ANYCHAIR YOGA

Anychair

YOGA

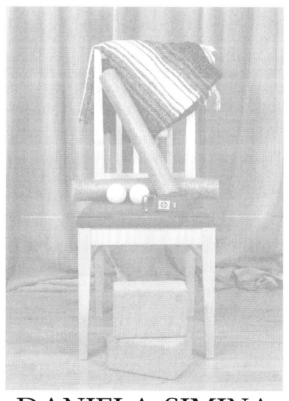

DANIELA SIMINA

ISBN: 1468150944

ISBN-13: 978-1468150940

Built upon holistic principles, the material presented in this book is intended as self-help for people who want to better their wellbeing by taking responsibility for their health. The information in this book is not meant for diagnosis or treatment for any medical condition. The author and publisher are not liable for any use or misuse of this material.

Acknowledgements

Heartfelt thanks to Graham Fowler, Director of Peachtree Yoga Center, who has played the essential role in my growth as a yoga teacher. Many thanks to Ursula Nix, Betsy Blount, Seth Adams, and to all the teachers at Peachtree Yoga Center for sharing with me their friendship and knowledge. I thank my students, as they've been my inspiration. I've learned from them as much as they've learned from me.

I would like to thank my husband, Marin Simina, whose work as photographer, designer and editor was essential for this book to come to life. I thank him for his support, for the long hours spent in the painstaking process of editing, and for his unwavering belief in me.

My gratitude goes to Melita Lawson, Land Fitness Coordinator at the Alpharetta YMCA, for her continuous support and encouragement. I want to thank Carol Berg, Terrie Russel, Janice Ramirez, Paula Philips Marrotte, and to all my friends who planted in my mind and in my heart the seed of this book.

Foreword

Thankfully, more and more people are taking responsibility for their own health. And we all know that a consistent and complete exercise program is one of the vital keys to the attainment and maintenance of good health.

From the good fortune of having Daniela Simina on teaching staff at my yoga center, I know that Daniela is a virtual storehouse of knowledge about health, and one of the most conscientious, knowledgeable, and creative yoga teachers I have ever met.

The practice of hatha yoga exercises, or asanas, has been rediscovered as uniquely suited to a variety of lifestyles. Millions of people are now enjoying a new lease on life from attending regular classes in yoga centers around the country.

But as wonderful as yoga is, if you don't do it, it won't work. So what about the many people who are unable to attend classes, due to physical limitation or logistical problems? Anychair Yoga fulfills the need to get started. Wherever you find yourself, whether in your home or at the office, there is always a chair. And wherever you can sit, you can benefit hugely from this book.

This jewel of a book holds the key to more strength, vitality and radiance, a healthy body, and a happy mind.

Graham Fowler, E-RYT 500
Founder/Director, Peachtree Yoga Center
Atlanta, Georgia

Preface

The concept behind *Anychair Yoga* is the following: there are people out there who need a yoga practice coming to them, because it is not always easy for them to go out for a yoga practice.

Over the past several years I came across a lot of people asking to be introduced to yoga, attracted by the benefits they heard such practice bestows upon one's body and mind. I brim with excitement whenever I receive such requests. As a yoga teacher, nothing brings me more joy then guiding people on this path. But among those expressing interested in yoga, one group got my attention in particular. People in this group had a common denominator, translated as pain, inflammation, poor balance, very limited flexibility, and no muscle strength. The perspective of being helpful to them seemed wonderful as I could understand how greatly beneficial yoga was in their case. But how should I guide through a physical yoga practice someone who can hardly move, can only stand up briefly, cannot walk without help, cannot fold forward, cannot lift the arms overhead, cannot twist, cannot get on the knees, and cannot get down on the floor, or if it gets down on the floor is unable to get up again?

I started to think of a way of practicing that addresses all concerns I heard those people expressing. I was looking for some prop, some "place" higher then the bare ground, something they could sit and get up easily from, something they could hold on when standing, something they have at home so they can practice without having to travel to a studio every day, something like…a chair! The next step was to look at different poses, and adapt them to fit a chair-based practice. The number one concern was how to adapt the poses still preserving the benefits of the standard, non-modified versions, while reducing intensity and providing additional support.

As the program outline was coming together, I realized that there's a far broader population that can benefit from it. I asked myself "What about people working in an office environment?" They spend a lot of time seated in a chair. Driving to a yoga studio at the end of the workday is often out of questions under the circumstances. The one thing omnipresent in an office environment, besides the computer is...a chair! There are simple yet efficient poses and breathing exercises helpful to manage stress and boost energy, which can be done on a chair. So, bringing yoga in the office is not just helpful, but also possible.

The aim of this program is to offer exposure to a well-balanced yoga practice, not just to some light stretches and moderate toning exercises. Consequently, breathing and relaxation techniques are presented in this book. The benefits of the postures are explained in relationship to anatomy and physiology, and detailed guidance is provided to maximize efficiency. To address all levels ability, several option are offered for a single pose, whenever suitable.

Many people understand they would greatly benefit from undertaking a consistent yoga practice. However, despite awareness, not everybody take this step, and even fewer would stick with such a practice over time. Knowing is different from actually doing it. What separates one group from another is motivation. Motivation is necessary to undertake the program, and even more motivation is needed to commit to it long enough to rip the benefits. The last chapter in this book makes suggestions about getting on track and getting back on track whenever getting off it because of adverse circumstances.

Last but not least, the final chapter in the book offers some ideas on how to maximize the benefits of your practice. Yoga is about living life in a holistic manner. This program aims at fostering wellbeing through integrating many components, which are vital to life itself such as movement, breathing, ability to relax, food, and water. The quality of food, water and lifestyle has been analyzed with the intent to provide information to be used in support to your quest for a higher quality of your life.

May the information presented in this book contribute to your good health and happiness!

Contents

1 Introduction

1.1 Who should care about a chair-based yoga practice

Anychair Yoga is a chair-based practice suitable for a wide variety of people ranging from the very fit to those with limited moving ability due to injury or other circumstances, such as being confined in the office or at home for a long time. Remaining active while confined to a chair or bed is really important since physical activity, even light, maintains proper blood flow and oxygenation in the body. During physical activity, even light, the brain receives more oxygen and this helps maintain focus, stay alert, eliminate feeling tired, and therefore being more productive while at work. Low impact yoga postures combined with breathing techniques promote release of serotonin, the neurotransmitter responsible for feeling relaxed and happy.

Awareness is the key ingredient for a successful practice (Schiffman, 1996). You should be one hundred percent present while practicing. Close the eyes whenever you deem it as possible and feel the slightest changes occurring into the body with the variation in alignment or deepening of the breath. This is how you develop body awareness. Don't allow any "to do list" run through your mind while engaged with your routine. Whenever you find yourself distracted redirect the attention back to the breath and back to the practice. Input equals output. The attention and dedication you put in shapes the result of your effort. Practicing without awareness deprives you of a rich experience and diminishes benefits.

The program described in this book goes beyond just using a chair as an aid for some stretches. Yoga is about bringing things together, and making them work in synergy. As the word synergy suggests, this program aims at fostering wellbeing at very deep levels by bringing together the tangible and the less tangible aspects of a human being into a cohesive, gentle, yet powerful practice. Standard yoga poses encountered in a regular mat-based practice have been adapted to fit the needs of people for whom such a practice is not an option. For more extensive use of props, refer to (Iyengar, 2001) and (Laseter, 1995). The selected breathing techniques are among the most widespread in yoga, and stood the proof of time as far as safety and efficiency concerns (Iyengar, 2005). Guided relaxation is becoming increasingly more popular, as more evidence about its positive impact on human physiology is piling up. More and more psychologist, psychiatrists, and physiologists recommend various relaxation techniques as part of stress management, pain management, and general wellness programs. The guided relaxation presented in this book is presented in steps easy to follow and is intended to complement and enhance the more physical part of the practice.

Anychair Yoga is for everybody. It addresses the needs of people spending long ours in the office, on long airplane travels, of those recovering recovery after brain surgery or other conditions where the sense of balance and coordination has been affected. It is for seniors as well as for athletes temporarily limited by injury. It can be used as an aid, to facilitate recovery from sport injuries and similar conditions that make locomotion and/or standing difficult. People can preserve flexibility and range of motion when temporary immobilized by injury or circumstances through remaining active at the low impact and steady pace of this program.

Anychair Yoga is not exclusively designed special population, but it is for anybody with a taste for trying something new. This program works thoroughly into your body by means of posture, breathing and guided relaxation techniques.

...And why chair yoga? Chairs are versatile yoga props and almost always at hand. Often times you don't even need to look specifically for a chair because you may be already sitting on one! And if you've been sitting on a chair for a long time, with your back, neck and hips feeling increasingly stiffer and numb, getting fidgety, with an irresistible urge to move around, well then you are in the right place at the right time for Anychair Yoga! You just need motivation and goal clarity to pursue your practice.

1.2 Internet Q/A and discussions

A Google group called *Anychair Yoga* was created for the readers of this book. Members can ask the author questions, share their experience and discuss the material presented in the book. The group's Internet address is: *http://groups.google.com/group/anychairyoga.*

1.3 Motivation, goals and persistence

To be successful in any endeavor, including learning and mastering the material presented in *Anychair Yoga*, one needs the ability to set up goals, plan how to achieve them, and have the discipline to follow these plans. Brian Tracy (Tracy, 2003) suggests writing down your goals regularly. We can start by writing hundred goals, which may help tremendously in clarifying priorities, understanding relationships among goals and why we want to pursue them. This helps in building the motivation required for being successful in our yoga program. As a next step, we can follow Brian Tracy's advice: choose one of the top goals and find twenty ways to achieve it. This provides an incredible exercise for creativity, since finding the last five ways can be very challenging. In the case of your yoga program, it may help you to transform the suggested programs in your own personalized creations. In turn, this will help build the motivation to pursue the programs. It may take three to six months to reap the benefits of pursuing your practice, so building a strong motivation and developing plans to achieve your goals is essential for your success.

1.4 A few safety considerations

Choose a sturdy chair that won't give way under your weight. Stability of the chair you use for practice is very important, therefore no rolling chairs, three legged chairs or anything other then a simple four legged chair with back support. If an office chair is the only one you have, lock the roles and check for stability before starting the practice.

Use for your practice a non-skid surface. This is especially important for standing poses. Take off your shoes and socks. In seated positions, shoes interfere with the ability to relax the feet, hindering blood circulation and creating excessive heat. In standing poses, shoes interfere not only with the ability to relax your feet but also with the proper positioning and alignment of the whole body compromising the quality of the practice. Wearing socks may work for seated poses, but they slide and twist around the feet in standing poses with a negative impact on proper feet positioning and stability.

1.5 Props

You may need few props (Figure 1) besides the chair you are using for the practice:

- 2-4 foam yoga blocks (a stack of old thick books could replace 2 of the blocks, the ones you use to put your feet on)

- One blanket or beach towel;

- Yoga strap or anything that can be used as a substitute, such as a belt;

- One beach noodle cut in thirds (you'll decide about the length of the pieces after reading the "Tennis ball or foam roll massage" section) or foam rolls such those used for myofascial release. You can purchase the foam rolls in stores selling sport article.

- Tennis ball

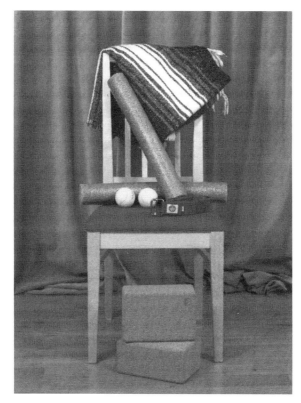

Figure 1: Props

1.6 Use this book to design your own practice

The book has sections on: Seated Poses, *Standing Poses, Restorative Poses, Guided Relaxation, Breathing Practice, and Leverage Your Potential.*

• Start your practice with 5-10 cycles of *complete breathing* described in the Breathing Practice chapter.

• Select three to five poses from each of the *Seated* and *Standing Poses* sections.

- Continue with about five minutes or more of one of the following: *complete breathing, step breathing,* or *alternate nostril breathing.*

- Add one *restorative pose.*

- Do the *guided relaxation.* Get familiar in advance with this part of the practice; learn few key points by heart.

- End with the *Deep Resting Pose.*

1.7 Sample practice

1   *Complete breathing* x 10 (see *Section 6.3*)

2   Seated *Side neck stretches* holding 5 breath cycles per each side (see *Section 2.4*)

3   Sliding the chin over the imaginary tennis ball exercise x5 (see *Section 2.6*)

4   *Cat arch cat lift* (see *Section 2.13*)

5   *Seated twists with crossed legs* (see *Section 2.19*). Hold each side for 5-7 breath cycles. Optional: you can do breathing with lengthened exhale while holding the twist.

6   *Wide legs seated position* (see *Section 2.24*)

7   *Pigeon* (see *Section 2.26*)

8   Transition from sitting to standing (see *Section 3.1*) up to 12 repetitions.

9   *Mountain pose* (see *Section 3.2*)

10 *Warrior 1* (see *Section 3.11*)

11 *Triangle* (see *Section 3.13*)

12 *Warrior 3* (see *Section 3.12*)

13 *Upward facing dog* (see *Section 3.5*)

14 *Downward facing dog* (see *Section 3.4*)

15 *Supported side bend,* (see *Section 4.2*) 7-10 breaths per side.

16 Seated upright with back unsupported: alternate nostril breathing (see *Section 6.7*) 2 min.

17 Sit in *Deep resting pose* (see *Section 4.3*) for the *Guided relaxation* (see *Section 5*).

18 Remain in the *Deep resting pose* for another 5-10 min.

2 Seated Poses

2.1 Why proper alignment is important

The human spine has several functions among which: protecting the spinal cord and the nerves associated with it, supporting the body in upright position, and allowing for flexibility. The spine has 5 natural curvatures. Their role is to make the spine strong and flexible so it can accomplish its functions. Improper sitting or standing positions lead to alteration of the spine curvatures. Overtime, postural deviations will occur and ultimately result in stiffness, back pain and loss of the spine's ability to perform its role (Coulter, 2001).

Prolonged slouching on a sofa or sitting with a rounded back and shoulders, and with the chin jotted forward can lead to a condition named kyphosis, which is a curving of the spine that causes the back to round excessively. Sitting with uneven hips, carrying heavy bags on the shoulder, or standing with the weight unevenly distributed can be factors contributing to scoliosis, which is a deviation of the spine side to side.

Weak abdominal muscles and/or excessive weight with most of the fat being stored on the abdomen may cause a protruding gut. When these combine with tight hamstrings and tight lower back muscles they lead to the occurrence of lordosis, which is an excessive arching of the lumbar curvature.

All these conditions cause significant overall discomfort, can become very painful, impairing therefore the body's ability to move and function. If neglected, they worsen in time. It is challenging to sit upright with your back unsupported over extended periods of time, but your ability to sit properly will improve as your back muscles strengthen, the muscles in your abdomen get stronger, and your hamstrings and hip flexors gain more flexibility.

2.2 Practicing proper alignment while seated on the chair

Benefits

Learning to sit erect and unsupported strengthens the back muscles, which is essential for proper spine alignment. Correct alignment facilitates breath and fends of pain resulting from unnecessary muscle tension.

Technique

Start seated on the chair with your back supported yet straight. If the soles of your feet are not completely flat on the ground use yoga blocks, a couple of thicker books or whatever you have at hand to prop up your feet. Adjust the height of your props so your thighs are parallel to the floor or very slightly lower then parallel to the floor. Positioning the legs this way allows you to slide back and sit closer to the chair's back support without having slouch in order to reach. Keep the hands resting on the lap and the shoulder relaxed.

- Pay attention to the pelvis, making sure the weight is evenly distributed on both sitting bones.

- Draw in slightly from about two inches bellow your navel to gently engage your abdominal muscles and avoid your pelvis to tilt forward too far, thus exaggerating the lumbar curve in an unwanted way.

- Lift the breastbone slightly to lift the rib cage and engage the upper back muscles.

- Feel your shoulder blades grounded into your back without stiffening the shoulders. If the shoulder blades are winged, gently guide them in the desired direction toward your back without squeezing aggressively your upper back muscles.

- Draw the back of your skull toward the wall behind you, just a little bit and notice how this simple and small adjustment engages your neck muscles and aligns your cervical spine.

- Keep your jaw parallel to the ground, keep your mouth closed without clenching the teeth, and relax your face muscles.

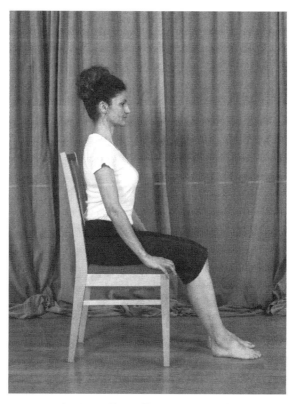

Figure 2: Sited with proper alignment

- Breathe fully but without strain and feel every inhale lengthening your spine. Feel your back muscles at work, slightly engaged but without clenching.

- Practice proper alignment first with your back supported, then gradually wean yourself off the support. Increase gradually the amount of time spent with your back unsupported and in proper alignment. Learn to sit properly weather your back is supported or not, and what's more important, take this practice with you at all times and in every place: at the table, in the office, in front of the TV or at the movies. Perseverance pays off!

2.3 Neck Exercises

Stiff neck muscles may cause a lot of problems ranging from limited mobility of the cervical spine to tension headaches. Weak neck muscles are unable to properly support the head and cause alteration of the cervical spine curvature resulting in discomfort or pain. Hence the importance of both stretching and toning the neck muscles
All the following neck exercises help stretching neck muscles and alleviate tension related pain. They strengthen the neck muscles so they can better support the cervical spine in proper alignment. These exercises are gentle enough to be accessible to every level but very efficient.

2.4 Neck side stretch

Benefits

The *Neck side stretch* emphasizes lengthening of the muscles situated laterally in the neck and helps developing more flexibility in the cervical spine through lateral flexion.

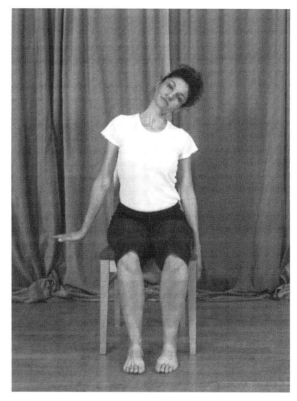

Figure 3: Neck side stretch

Technique

- Start seated with a straight back (unsupported, if possible).

- Stretch your right arm laterally to the right, and about 3 inches below the shoulder level.

- Flex your wrist, pulling the back of the hand toward you.

- Press away through the heel of the hand.

- Tilt the head to the right, keeping the left ear in line with the left shoulder.

- You may keep the position stationary, or you can make very small movements (the range of eights of an inch) to find the right spot.

The right spot is the one where you get a pleasant feeling stretch with no sharp pain or other significant discomfort.

- Hold for 5 to 7 breath cycles for each side.

2.5 The Giraffe

Benefits

This exercise has a traction-like effect. It gradually lengthens the cervical spine and diminishes compression on the disks.

Technique

- Start seated with the back straight (unsupported, if possible).

- Keep the shoulder blades flat against the back and reaching toward your back pockets.

- Reach the top of your head as high as you possible can while pressing the shoulders down.

- Tilt the head side to side with very small movements, aiming to lengthen the neck more each time you tilt.

- The sensation you should create is that of your neck getting longer and longer, like a giraffe's neck.

- Do it for about 2 minutes.

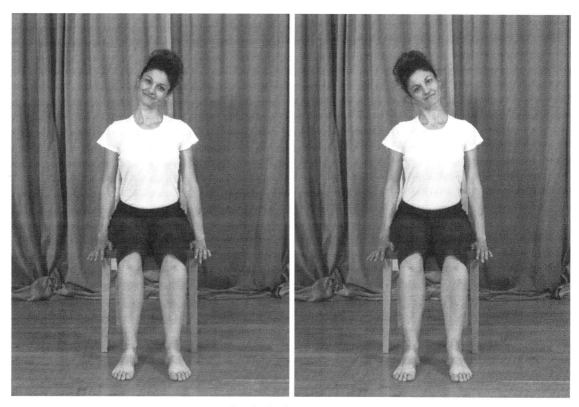

Figure 4: Head tilt left and right (the Giraffe)

2.6 Slide the Chin Over the Tennis Ball

Benefits

This exercise stretches the back of the neck, and opens the spaces between the vertebrae reducing compression on the intervertebral disks.

Technique

- Start seated with the back straight (unsupported, if possible).

- Keep the shoulder blades flat against the back and reaching toward your back pockets.

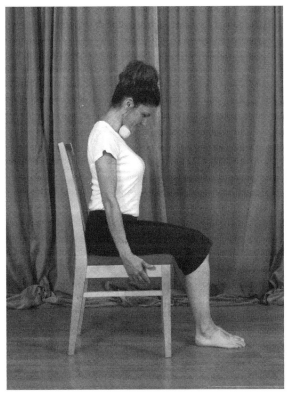

Figure 5: Slide the chin over the tennis ball

- Reach the top of your head as high as you possible can while pressing the shoulders down.

- Hold a tennis ball in front of your throat, or you can imagine a tennis ball being placed in front of your throat.

- In order to slide the chin over the real or imaginary ball, reach first your chin forward lengthening you neck then lower the chin toward the chest passed the ball.

- Hold the stretch for 3 -5 breaths cycles.

- Do the whole thing in reverse.

- Repeat the whole exercise 3 -5 times.

2.7 Neck Half Roles

Benefits

This exercise improves flexibility in the cervical spine and stretches the muscles of the back and sides of the neck reducing tension in the neck. It warms up the neck muscles and helps lubricating the joints. It releases tension and improves circulation in the neck, reduces inflammation and helps preventing the reoccurrence of tension headache.

Technique

- Start seated with the back straight (unsupported, if possible).

- Keep the shoulders away from the ears without stiffening.

- Drop the chin to the chest relaxing the neck muscles.

- Slowly, role your head to the right until you get the right ear over your right shoulder.

- Slowly, role your head to the left until you get the left ear over your left shoulder.

- Pause along the way holding the stretch that's right on target.

- Do 5-7 cycles, counting one motion right to left and left to right as one cycle.

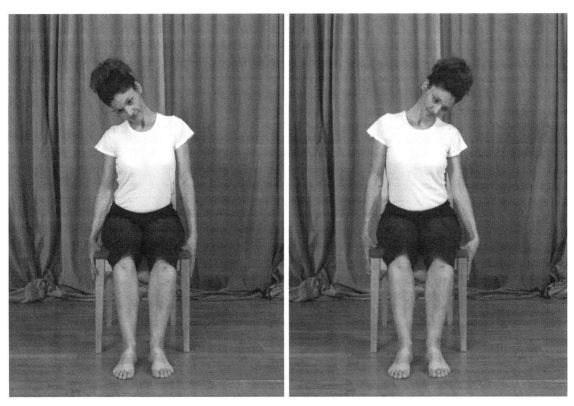

Figure 6: Neck half roles

2.8 Using Gentle Pressure

You can use gentle pressure to release tension in large muscle group large groups by rolling over a tennis ball or foam roll. You can make your own rolls by cutting a foam noodle into 3 pieces.

2.9 Massaging the upper back

Benefits

This exercise uses gentle pressure to release tension and pain in the back muscles.

Technique

- Place the tennis ball between your shoulder blades and squeeze it gently against the back of the chair.

- Move slowly the ball side to side by rolling your back over it. You can make circular motions if you can secure the ball preventing it from popping out.

- Do the same with the shoulder blades, first the right then the left.

Be careful! Don't put too much pressure and don't spend more then 1 minute per each section you are massaging. Overdoing it may cause tissues to bruise and create even more pain! You may need some help to place a tennis ball between your upper back and the chair. A foam roll placed vertically against your upper back in the area you intend to massage is easier to use in this case. You won't be able to massage circularly with the foam roll and the sensation is usually less intense, but it is easier to maneuver then the ball. Use the same caution as you would with the tennis ball: avoid excessive pressure and limit the use to one minute or slightly less per session.

2.10 Gluteus massage

Benefits

This exercise uses gentle pressure to release tension and pain in the rear end muscles.

Technique

- Sit on top of a foam roll long enough to accommodate the gluteus on both right and left sides.

- Hold on the seat partly supporting the body and assist movement.

- Roll back and forth for 1-2 minutes.

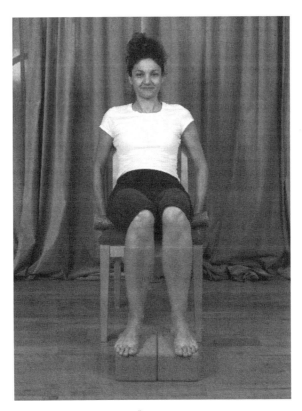

Figure 7: Gluteus massage

2.11 Hamstrings massage

Benefits

This exercise uses gentle pressure to release tension and pain in the rear end muscles. Releasing tension in the hamstring allows sitting with the back in proper alignment and bending forward without straining the lower back.

Technique

- Sit with the back of your leg on top of a piece of noodle.

- Hold on the seat partly supporting the body and assist movement.

- Roll back and forth for 1-2 minutes for each side.

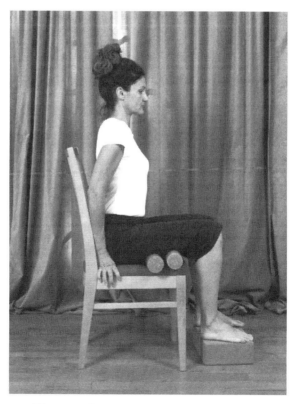

Figure 8: Hamstrings massage

2.12 Massage the soles of the feet

Benefits

This exercise helps alleviate pain associated with plantar fasciitis; it provides a calming and relaxing foot massage.

Technique

- Sit on the chair with a straight back.

- Place the right foot on a piece of noodle.

- Hold on the seat to get a sense of increased stability.

- Role the noodle, back and forth, with your foot insisting on the spots that feel tenser.

- You can do up to 5 minutes for each side and you can use a tennis ball or a golf ball instead of a beach noodle.

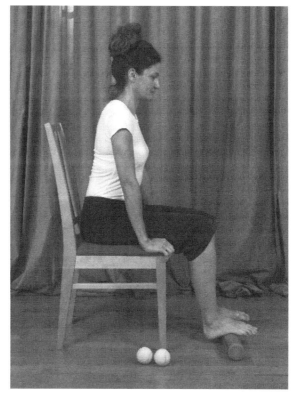

Figure 9: Massage the soles of the feet

2.13 Cat tuck and Cat lift

Benefits

This exercise stretches and tones muscles in the whole back, in particular those muscles associated with flexion and extension of the spine. It makes the vertebral column more flexible, works toward correcting postural imbalances, and gently stimulates the central nervous system since the major nerves run longitudinally through the backbone. It is a good warm up exercise preparing the back, chest and shoulder muscle for more engaging poses.

Technique

- Sit with your back unsupported, holding on the seat.

- Exhale and round the back, dropping the chin toward the chest and tucking the tailbone. Pull slightly the seat toward you to enhance the rounding of the spine.

- The space in between the vertebrae opens up stretching the intertwining muscles and releasing the disks form compression.

- Inhale and arch out the back by lifting the breastbone and sticking the tailbone out. Gently press the back of your skull toward the wall behind you. Pull the seat toward you to assist the arching and to enhance the stretch in the chest muscles.

- One rounding of the back (cat arch) and one arching out of the back (cat lift) is one cycle. Do 10-15 cycles.

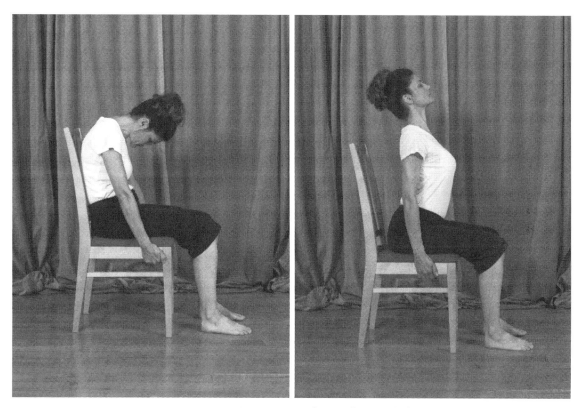

Figure 10: Cat tuck and Cat lift

2.14 Shoulders shrugs and presses

Benefits

This very simple practice tones and stretches the some muscles associated with the shoulders and upper back. It helps lubricating the shoulder joint, which makes motion smoother and less painful wherever inflammatory conditions such as arthritis exist. It helps developing flexibility in the shoulder, therefore increasing the range of motion.

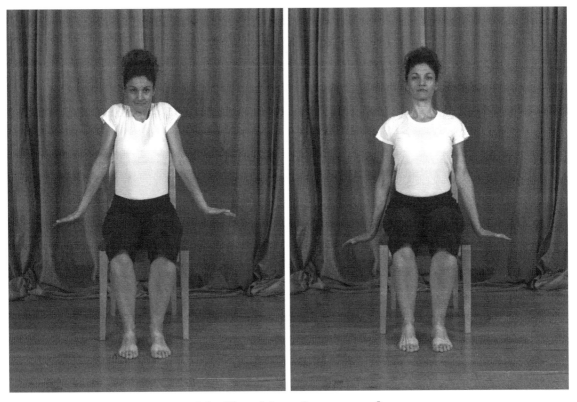

Figure 11: Shoulder shrugs and presses

Technique

- Sit with the back unsupported with the arms by your sides.

- Bend the wrists with the fingers pointing out.

- Inhale and shrug the shoulders.

- Exhale and press the shoulders down. Feel as if you want to push the floor away with the heels of your hands.

- Repeat 10 times.

2.15 Shoulders circles with a strap

Benefits

This exercise is primarily designed to increase flexibility in the shoulder joint by stretching the muscles associated with it. It helps improve the range of motion in the shoulder joint.

Technique

- Start seated with the back unsupported.

- Hold a yoga strap or a towel with your both hands, palms facing down; the distance in between your hands should be significantly wider then your shoulders.

- Stretch the strap by pulling at its ends without creating excessive tension in your arms. Keep the arms in front of you in a low position where the strap is barely touching your legs.

- Inhale while moving the straight arms overhead and exhale as you lower them behind you.

- Undo, moving the arms in reverse. Inhale while lifting the arms from behind you up overhead, and exhale as you lower the arms back in front of you in the starting position.

- If you can't get the arms behind you allow more distance in between your hands.

- Start with a wider grip and then, as your shoulders warm up you can reposition your hands slightly closer.

- Do 5-8 cycles.

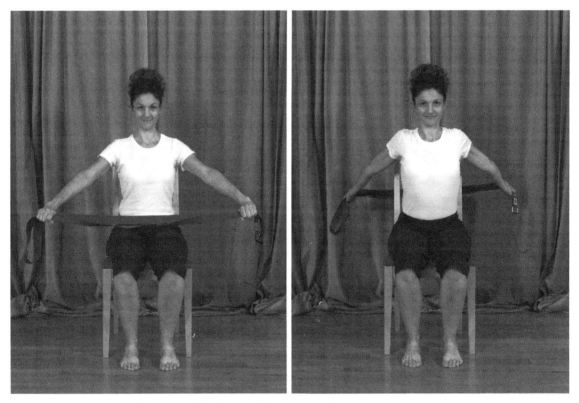

Figure 12: Shoulders circles with a strap

2.16 Wrists: toning and stretching

Benefits

This exercise tones and stretches the wrist joint. Lack of tone and flexibility in the wrist may lead to pain and discomfort. Certain conditions such as carpal tunnel syndrome benefit greatly from exercises that tone and stretch the wrist joint and the muscles associated with it.

Technique

- From sitting with the back straight, lift the arms in front of you with the elbows bent to avoid unnecessary tension to build in the arms.

- Open and close the hands. Do it 7-10 times slow squeezing the fists when closing the hands, and stretching the fingers wide when you open your palms. Do it again 7-10 times as fast as you can, emphasizing just speed.

2.17 Toning the arms and chest muscles

Benefits

This exercise strengthens the arms and the chest muscles in a gentle manner setting up the ground for more intense activities. A lifestyle lacking physical activity lead to denegation of muscle tissue in the arms and chest and chest. Strong arms and chest muscles are necessary to successfully carry on every day activities without developing inflammation and pain in the shoulders, elbows, and wrists. Strong chest muscles are an important prerequisite for good posture.

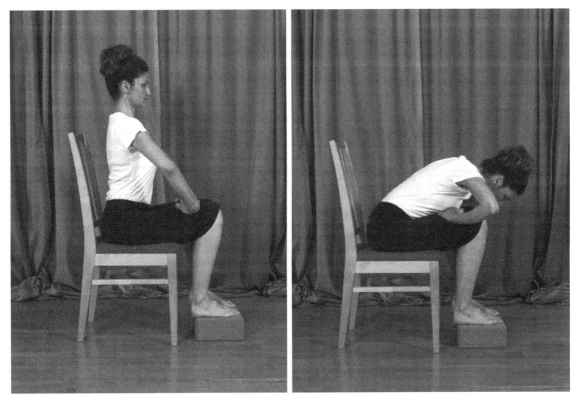

Figure 13: Toning arms and chest muscles

Technique

- Sit with the feet propped up on blocks or on a stack of books.

- Place palms on the knees with fingers covering the kneecaps.

- Slide the heels of your hands forward enough to create an angle wider then 90 degrees between your forearm and the back of your hand.

- Keep hands firm but relaxed.

- Engage the abdominal muscles by slightly pulling from about two inches below the navel.

- Lean forward transferring as much weight to your arms as it feels comfortable.

- Inhale as you flex the elbows in a push-up like motion getting the chest as close to the legs as you can.

- Exhale while you press back up.

- You will engage primarily the chest muscles by allowing the elbows to move out to the sides as you flex the arms.

- Repeat.

- You will engage primarily the triceps by keeping the elbows close to the rig cage as you flex the arms.

- Do 5 -10 repetitions of each kind.

2.18 Twists with parallel legs

Benefits

Twists are important for a number a reasons. They relax and stretch the back muscles and the spine, gently massage the internal organs assisting digestion and elimination processes. Major nerves are housed in the spine so twists act in a gentle way upon the nervous system as well. Parallel leg twist is indicated for people having hip replacement where bringing the thighbone across the midline is not indicated.

Technique

- Seat upright with the feet parallel, about hips distance apart.

- Keep the lower legs perpendicular to the ground (your knees should be over the ankles). Maintain the thighs parallel with each other and avoid the knees spilling out to the sides.

- Take the left arm across and place the left hand on the outside of your right thigh, holding at your leg.

- Place the right hand behind you, close to the base of the spine, with fingers pointing out.

- Start twisting to the right. Progress gently into the twist, lengthening the spine on the inhale and twisting a bit deeper on the exhale.

- Complete the twist by turning the head to the right as far as comfortable for your neck.

- Do about 10 breath cycles for each side.

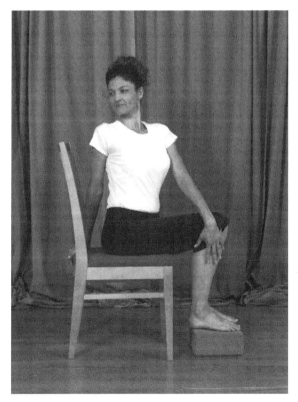

Figure 14: Twists with parallel legs

2.19 Cross-legged twist

Benefits

This twist works more intense on the outer thighs muscles. By grounding the sitting bones and maintaining the pelvis leveled the lower back muscles and the gluteus experience a deeper stretch. This twist is not indicated for people with hip replacement

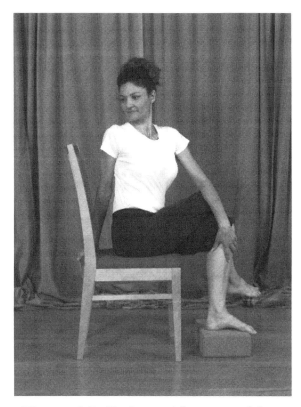

Figure 15: Twists with crossed legs

Technique

- Seat upright with the feet parallel, close together.

- Keep the lower legs perpendicular to the ground (your knees should be over the ankles).

- Cross your right leg over the left, getting the right knee on top of the left.

- Take the left arm across and place the left hand on the outside of your right thigh, holding at your leg.

- Place the right hand behind you, close to the base of the spine, with fingers pointing out.

- Start twisting to the right. Progress gently into the twist, lengthening the spine on the inhale and twisting a bit deeper on the exhale.

- Complete the twist by turning the head to the right as far as comfortable for your neck.

- Do about 10 breath cycles for each side.

2.20 Prayer twist

Benefits

This twist engages the upper back and chest muscles a little more then the versions mentioned previously. The top shoulder turns open getting the associated muscles to contract while the palms pressing against each other engage the chest muscles. By getting leverage from the arm bone positioned across the thigh one can deepen the twist and get a more pronounced stretch in the back muscles. It is important to maintain the knees even while twisting to keep the sacroiliac joint in alignment.

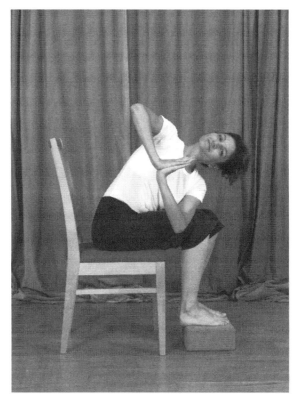

Figure 16: Prayer twist

Technique

- Seat upright with the feet parallel, close together, each foot on a block.

- Keep the lower legs perpendicular to the ground (your knees should be over the ankles).

- Bring the hands in front of the chest with palms together and elbows wide. The forearms should be in line.

- Twist to the right and bring the left elbow across the left leg, with hands together and forearms in line.

- Keep the spine long and flex the torso forward as deep as it feels comfortable.

- Keep the neck neutral or turn the face up if it feels good in your neck.

- Do about 5-10 breath cycles for each side.

2.21 Boat pose

Benefits

This pose targets the abdominals in particular, but it also works on strengthening the hip flexors and the lower back muscles. Strong abdominals protect the lower back from injury and contributes to proper body alignment and a healthy spine. Practices meant to strengthen the abdominals provide a gentle massage to the internal organs with positive effects on digestion and detoxification. Strong abdominal muscles also provide better protection for the internal organs preventing them to prolapse and help recovery when the condition is already present.

Technique

- Seat on the chair slightly farther away from the back support. Initially the back is upright and unsupported.

- Place the feet on blocks, about pelvis distance apart, with the knees tracking the ankles.

- Start engaging the abdominals by drawing in from right bellow the navel; support this action by slightly tucking the tailbone under. At this point the pelvis should tilt slightly toward the chair's back creating a rounding sensation in the lower back.

- Maintain the chest open, don't round the upper back; it is only the lowest portion of your back that is rounding barely, due to the pelvic tilt. Preserve this alignment in the upper body as you lean back getting the shoulder blades to touch the chair back support.

- Lift the right foot of the block; you may just have the foot hovering or if you strong enough get it as high as you can. As you lift the foot of the block and lift further, maintain your awareness glued to the lower abdomen and lower back. Do not relax the drawing in of the navel or the tuck in the tailbone! If these areas relax the entire effort transfers to the lower back muscles resulting in unnecessary strain; in parallel, the strengthening action in the abdominals gets lost. The result of this posture is directly proportional to your degree of awareness, and not to how high you lift the legs.

- Hold the right foot up for 5-7 breaths cycles, lower it down without changing the position of the upper body, and then do the left leg.

- People with stronger abdominal muscles can take the challenge one step further.

- Seat on the chair slightly farther away from the back support. Initially the back is   upright and unsupported.

- Place the feet on blocks, about pelvis distance apart, with the knees tracking the ankles.

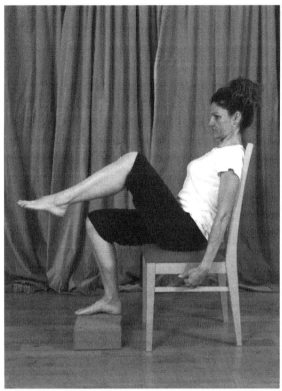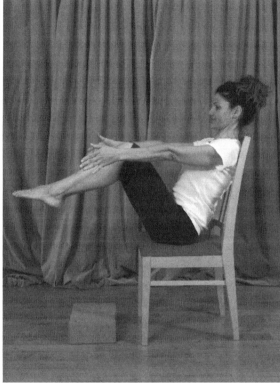

Figure 17: Boat pose

- Start engaging the abdominals by drawing in from right bellow the navel; support this action by slightly tucking the tailbone under. At this point the pelvis should tilt slightly toward the chair's back creating a rounding sensation in the lower back.

- Maintain the chest open, don't round the upper back; it is only the lowest portion of your back that is rounding barely, due to the pelvic tilt. Preserve this alignment in the upper body as you lean back getting the shoulder blades to touch the chair back support.

- Pick up your right foot, lift it about 6 inches above the blocks or higher, then lift the left foot as well. Same as specified above, do not relax the drawing in of the navel or the tuck in the tailbone! If these areas relax the entire effort transfers to the lower back muscles resulting in unnecessary strain; also, the strengthening action in the abdominals gets lost.

- You may hold on the chair for some extra support, or you may stretch the arms out to the sides or in front of you.

2.22 Side bending flow

Benefits

This flow sequence stretches the intercostal muscles enhancing the flexibility of the ribcage. Flexibility in these muscles is important since allows for deeper and more efficient breathing.

Technique

- Seat upright with the feet parallel, close together, each foot on a block.

- Keep the lower legs perpendicular to the ground (your knees should be over the ankles).

- Keep the pelvis level by avoiding excessive arching in the lower back or rounding in the upper back.

- Keep the right arm hanging down or rest the palm next to you on the chair seat.

- Lift the right arm overhead with the palm facing toward you. If lifting the arm overhead is not possible due to a physical limitation such as frozen shoulder only lift the arm parallel to the ground or keep the hand on your waist.

- Inhale and lengthen the body.

- Exhale and bend to the left. Go only as far as you can maintain both sitting bones evenly grounded on the chair.

- Mind your neck. If you have a neck condition preventing you from turning the face up, keep the neck neutral or look down. You can allow the head to hang, stretching the neck muscles.

- Inhale and lift the torso up to vertical.

- Change position of the arms, lowering the right and lifting the left.

- Exhale and bent to the right.

- Inhale lift all the way up.

- Do 5-10 cycles.

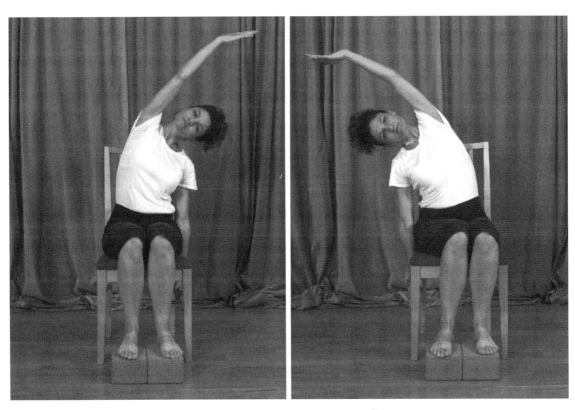

Figure 18: Side bending flow

2.23 Seated forward fold

Benefits

This pose stretches gently the lower back muscles, relaxes the shoulders and the neck muscles. In the deeper version the head is lower then the chest and because of this the brain benefits from an increased blood flow.

Technique

- For a small range of motion forward fold start with the feet on the floor or on a block.

- Keep the back straight.

- Place the feet together.

- Stretch the arms in front, then bend the arms and hold at the elbows.

- Flex torso forward until the forearms are supported on your legs.

- Relax the neck and allow your head to hang.

- Hold for 5 breath cycles or for as long as you wish.

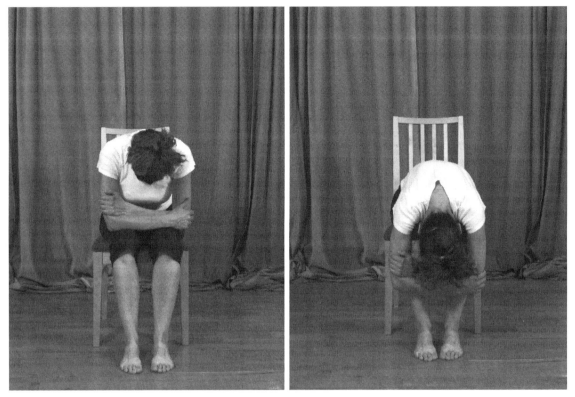

Figure 19: Seated forward fold

- For a deeper forward fold start with the feet on the floor.

- Keep the back straight.

- Hinge forward without holding the elbows.

- You can rest the hands on blocks (one block or several blocks, stacked) placed to give enough support to avoiding squeezing the chest against the legs.

- Relax the neck and allow your head to hang.

- Hold for 5 breath cycles or for as long as you wish.

2.24 Wide legs seated position

Benefits

This pose stretches the inner thighs muscles, and since involves sitting with the back unsupported it engages the core muscles to support the upright position.

Technique

- Sit upright with the back unsupported.

- Keep the pelvis leveled to the chair without arching or rounding the lower back. Have your weight evenly distributed on both sitting bones.

- You can have your feet on blocks if the knees are too low and you feel sliding forward off the chair.

- Spread the legs as wide as you can without altering the upper body alignment.

- Keep the arms relaxed on your legs or hold on the chair for an increased sense of stability. You may find that holding on the chair also assist your upright unsupported back position.

- Hold for about 10 -15 breaths cycles.

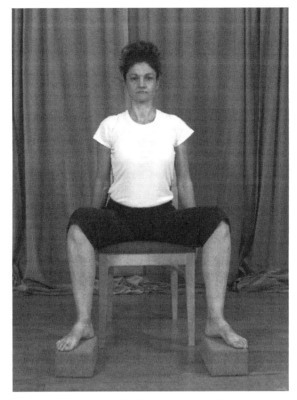

Figure 20: Wide legs seated position

2.25 Cobbler's pose on the chair

Benefits

This pose stretches the inner thighs and groin muscles.

Technique

- Start seated with the back supported and the feet very close together, raised on two or three stacked blocks.

- Keep the inner edges of your feet touching and drop the thighs open.

- Allow the inner thighs muscles to stretch gently under the action of your own leg's weight pulling out and downward.

- Hold for 10 breaths cycles or for as long as you wish.

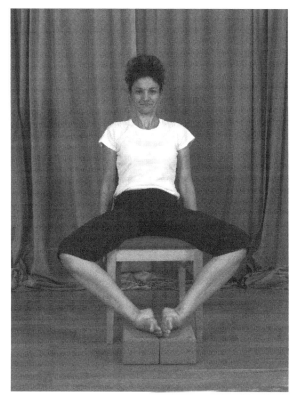

Figure 21: Cobbler's pose on the chair

2.26 Pigeon pose

Benefits

This pose is invaluable when it comes to stretching the outer thighs muscles such as the IT band and muscles located deeply in the rear end area such as the Piriformis.

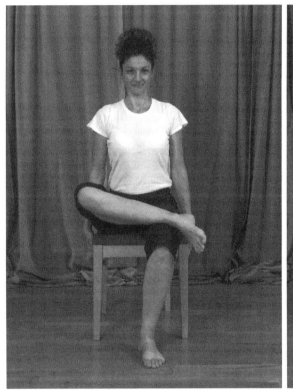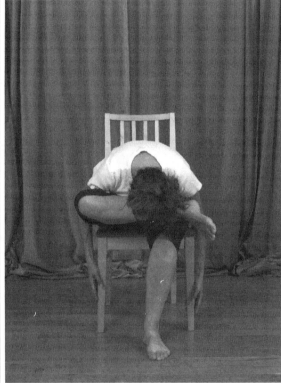

Figure 22: Pigeon pose

Technique

- Start seated with the back upright.

- Pick up your right leg and bring the ankle across your left knee.

- Lean forward to create just enough intensity in your right outer leg and the right side of the rear end. You can place a small pillow or folded blanket on your lap and use it for support. It is utmost important to be comfortable in the pose so you can relax and breath smoothly. Hold for 10 breath cycles or more.

- Do the other side.

3 Standing Poses

3.1 Relearning to transition from sitting to standing

There may be situations when moving from seated to a standing position is challenging. It is important to keep working on strengthening the legs so they can support the body while standing or walking.

Benefits

The following flow sequence done regularly improves balance, tones up the legs muscles, enhances blood flow in the legs, keep joints lubricated, preparing you for longer walks or longer time spent standing.

Technique

- Start seated on a chair with a second chair with its back support within reach. If a second chair is not at available you can use a tabletop or the wall for support. You should be able to place your hands on the support in front without stretching the arms completely.

- Set your feet parallel, about pelvis distance apart. A wider base will give your body more stability. As your practice progresses you'll be able to stand with the feet closer together. Keep your back upright, use the chair in front for support and get up to standing.

- Pause into a standing position. Perfect your alignment as follow described in *Mountain pose*, which is nothing but standing in proper alignment.

3.2 Mountain pose

Benefits

This pose teaches proper alignment which is very important for a healthy back. In the beginning you may need the additional support to stand up. With practice you will feel more confident and stable and your need for additional support will diminish.

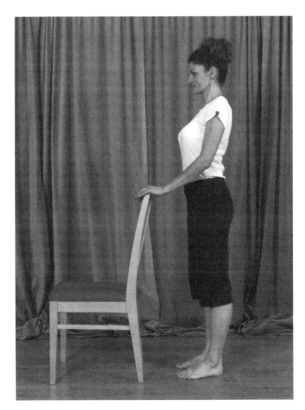

Figure 23: Mountain pose

Technique

- You just moved into standing holding on the back of the second chair, as described in the section above.

- Have your feet parallel, positioned about pelvis distance apart.

- Still holding on your support, ground your feet, spread the toes, engage slightly the front of the thighs muscles (you'll feel the knee cap lifting slightly), tone gently your rear end muscles (without squeezing excessively), and draw in slightly from about two inches below the navel.

- Lift the breastbone; keep the shoulders relaxed and the arms down by your sides. If your balance is uncertain, keep holding on the additional chair but don't clench your hands. Have your hands rather resting on the back of the addition chair instead of gripping.

- Energize slightly the arms just enough to feel a little bit of muscular engagement without stiffening.

- If you don't need additional support to stand up, then keep extend the arms along the body with the palms open, turning forward, with the fingers straight but not stiff. Lengthen the neck and keep the jaw parallel to the floor.

- Hold the pose for 7-10 breaths cycles allowing time for your body to memorize the feeling of being in correct alignment.

- You can sit back and stand up again. Start with one repetition, and progress to 10 -12 repetitions.

As this practice becomes easier, start doing it by breath: take one full inhale as you stand up, one full exhale as you sit down. Move with the breath but don't force any unnatural, strenuous breathing pattern. Start with the number of repetitions that feels comfortable and progress from there. As you feel this variation getting too easy, give up the additional support, transitioning from seated to standing and from standing to seat without any additional support.

3.3 Standing forward fold

Benefits

This is a pose where your head gets below the chest. Such poses facilitate blood flow to the brain and other vital organs in the upper body, increasing the oxygenation of those organs. Additionally, the Standing forward fold stretches the back of the legs and lower back muscles.

Technique

- Start standing in *Mountain pose* (see Figure 23) at about one, one and a half afoot in front of the chair, facing the seat.

- Inhale and lift the arms overhead.

- Exhale and fold forward, getting the hands on the seat with flat palms.

- Allow the arms to support the weight of the torso, still keeping some degree of softness in your shoulders, elbows and wrists. Don't lock in the elbows.

- Drop the head, softening the back of the neck muscles.

- Feel the back of your legs and the lower back muscles releasing tension with each exhale. As this happens, you may want to get deeper into the forward fold.

- If you are flexible enough, you can place your forearms on the seat.

- In time you may become able to bring the forehead to the seat.

- If you are new to yoga and uncomfortable being head down, start by holding this position for 3 breathe cycles. As you are getting increasingly comfortable about it, you can extend the time up to 10 breaths cycles.

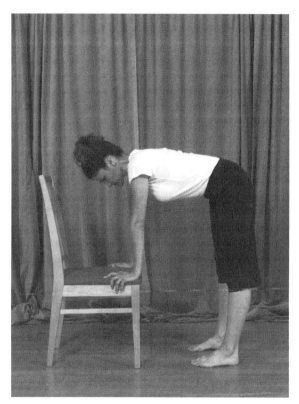

Figure 24: Standing forward fold

3.4 Downward facing dog

Benefits

This pose is a great shoulders opener, stretches the back of the legs, and neutralizes tension in the lower back.

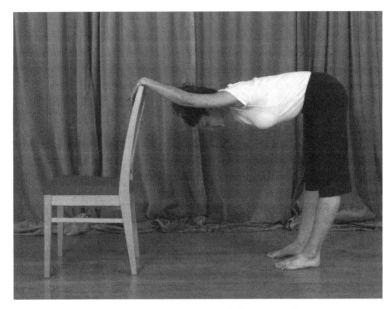

Figure 25: Downward facing dog 1

Technique

• Start standing in *Mountain pose* at about one and a half, two feet in behind the chair, facing the back support.

• Inhale and lift the arms overhead.

• Exhale and fold forward maintaining straight legs and straight back as you fold.

• Get the hands on top of the back support and hold on the chair without gripping.

- Allow the arms to support the weight of the torso keeping the shoulders relaxed.

- Keep the arms straight, but don't lock in the elbows.

- Drop the head, softening the back of the neck muscles.

- If you are really flexible and this position doesn't stretch you well enough, then do it with the hands on the seat instead. The overall body alignment stays the same, only your torso folds deeper. If doing the downward facing dog with hands on the seat variation make sure the arms are straight, otherwise your shoulder's won't get the same amount of stretching as in the first variation.

- Hold 5-10 breath cycles.

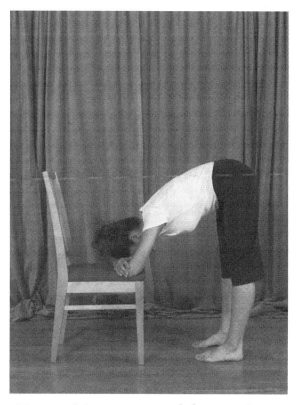

Figure 26: Downward facing dog 2

3.5 Upward facing dog

Benefits

This pose is a moderate backbend as well as a chest opener. It strengthens all the muscles associated with the spine and opens up the chest area.

Technique

- Start standing in *Mountain pose* (see Figure 23) behind the chair, facing the back support. Your body should be close enough to touch slightly the chair.

- Place the hands on the top of the back support.

- Tuck the tailbone and maintain the rear end muscles engaged to prevent overarching in the lower back.

- Lift the breastbone as you press the hands against the chair.

- Keep the shoulders away from the ears.

- Draw the shoulder blades down along the back.

- Focus on the space between the shoulder blades and feel as if your back were arching from that place.

- Lengthen the neck and glance up.

- Don't collapse into the lower back.

- Keep pushing away through your hands. Don't bend too far back griping at the back support. Don't use the chair as counterweight to keep you stable: you may fell back and pull the chair with you.

- Begin with 2-3 breaths cycles. As your practice progresses you may increase to 5 breaths cycles.

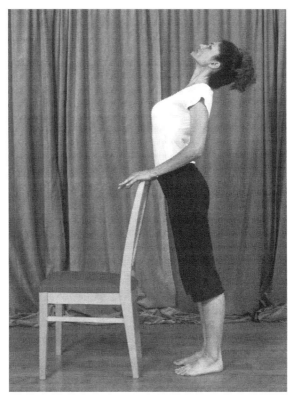

Figure 27: Upward facing dog

3.6 Chair pose

Benefits

Practiced regularly, the *Chair pose* (see Figure 29: Chair pose 2) strengthens the legs and core muscles. Strengthening the upper leg muscles in turn stabilizes the knee joint.

Technique

Based on the degree of strength, the pose can be approached in a number of ways. If the legs muscles are really weak with some degree of atrophy as a result of being immobilized for a long time, don't aim to get completely off the chair at first (see Figure 28: Chair pose 1). Start seated on the chair with the back upright and unsupported. Position the feet flat on the floor, about pelvis distance apart. The lower legs are perpendicular on the floor with the knees tracking the ankles.

- Place the hands on the chair close to you or on your thighs.

- Angle the torso slightly forward.

- Engage the abdominal muscles by drawing in the navel and slightly tucking the tailbone under. You may get the feeling that the pelvis is slightly tilting posteriorly.

- Press firmly the feet into the ground, and gradually engage the muscle in your legs and buttocks as if you want to get off the chair. This is not necessarily about transitioning into a standing position; it is about strengthening the legs through contracting the muscles during a weight bearing practice.

- Hold the contraction in your muscles for one or two breath cycles, making sure you don't hold the breath as well.

- Release and sit for a couple of breaths and reposition the body, getting ready to start again.

- Repeat the cycle of contracting-releasing the muscles for 5-10 times.

- In time you will move to the next level where you'll actually get off the chair completely.

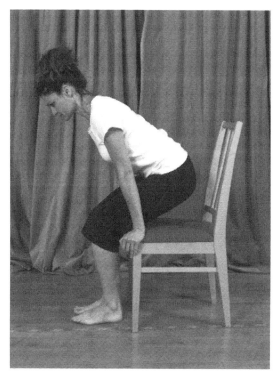

Figure 28: Chair pose 1

If your legs are strong enough to support standing and walking with minimal aid, you may start working at a different level of intensity then the one suggested above.

- Start seated on the chair with the back upright and unsupported. Position the feet flat on the floor, about pelvis distance apart. The lower legs are perpendicular on the floor with the knees tracking the ankles.

- Engage the abdominal muscles by drawing in the navel and slightly tucking the tailbone under. You may get a pronounced feeling that the pelvis is slightly tilting posteriorly.

- Place the hands on the chair close to you or on your thighs, or for more challenge get the arms straight in front of you and parallel to the floor.

- Press firmly the feet into the ground, and gradually engage the muscle in your legs and buttocks, get your rear end to hover above the chair, ending in a semi-squatting position.

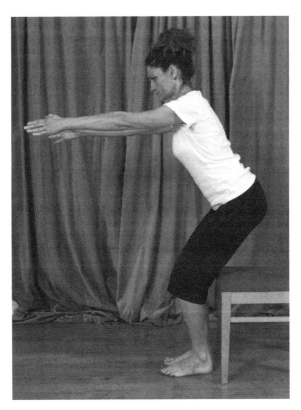

Figure 29: Chair pose 2

- The lower you remain, the more intense the pose becomes. If it feels like too much, get slightly higher in the pose by straightening the knees a little bit. As you do this, make sure the abdominal muscles remain engaged to protect the lower back; pay constant attention to the tuck of the tailbone and the navel drawing in. Don't hold the breath as you consciously engage the muscles.

- Hold the pose for as long as you deem necessary; it should feel challenging without feeling excessive or painful on any body part, especially on your knees or lower back.

- You may do 2-5 repetitions, allowing a couple of breath cycles in between for recovery.

There's a yet another way to approach the pose, meant for people with quite strong legs but who have a harder time balancing and maintaining the core muscles engaged while squatting, as required in Chair Pose (see Figure 30: Chair pose 3).

- Start standing about one foot, one foot and a half behind the chair, depending how long your arms are and how far forward you are going to angle the body. The feet are parallel and placed about pelvis distance apart for easier balance.

- Place the hands on the back of the chair keep the arms straight but do not lock in the elbows.

- Draw in from bellow the navel and slightly tuck the tailbone to engage the abdominal muscles. You should feel the pelvis slightly tilting toward the back. Breath naturally, without straining.

- Squat as you angle the torso forward. Maintain the weight predominantly on your heels.

- Go only as deep as you can maintain proper alignment: keep the back straight without arching, place the weight on the heels, keep the knees behind the toes even if not quite over the ankles, and the lower portion of the abdomen gently drawing in.

- Hold for as long as you want, aiming to create some degree of challenge but staying away from an edge that could lead to aggravation.

- You can do it just once or repeat it up to four times, resting for a couple of breaths in between repetitions.

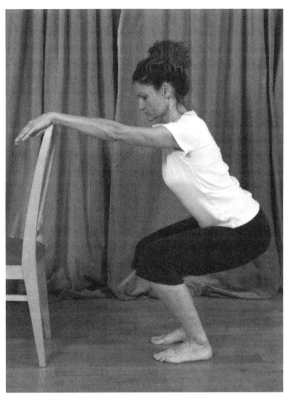

Figure 30: Chair pose 3

3.7 Chair pose with a block

Benefits

There is yet another approach to *Chair pose*, which is safe, gentle and challenging altogether (see Figure 31: Chair pose with a block 1). In addition to strengthening the front of the thighs and core muscles, placing the yoga block between the knees adds more intensity to the pose because it engages the inner thighs muscles more then the previous options. The higher the pressure applied to the block, the more intense is the effort required from the inner thighs muscles. Balancing in this pose is still easy despite the added intensity, since the distance between the feet doesn't change compared to the previous variations. Also, compressing the block between the knees while in the semi-squat position required by the Chair pose aligns the sacroiliac joint helping with pain management.

Technique

Based on the degree of leg strength, the pose can be approached in two ways. If the legs muscles are rather weak, you can approach the pose from a seated position (*Chair pose with a block 1*). Start seated on the chair with the back upright and unsupported. Position the feet flat on the floor, about pelvis distance apart. The lower legs are perpendicular on the floor with the knees tracking the ankles.

- Place the block between the knees.

- Place the hands on the chair close to you or on your thighs.

- Angle the torso slightly forward.

- Engage the abdominal muscles by drawing in the navel and slightly tucking the tailbone under. You may get the feeling that the pelvis is slightly tilting posteriorly.

- Press firmly the feet into the ground, and gradually engage the muscle in your legs and buttocks as if you want to get off the chair. This is not necessarily about transitioning into a standing position; it is about strengthening the legs through contracting the muscles during a weight bearing practice.

- Keep compressing the block weather you are hovering slightly above the chair or you are mostly seated.

- Hold the contraction in your muscles for one or two breath cycles, making sure you don't hold the breath as well.

- Release and sit for a couple of breaths and reposition the body, getting ready to start again.

- Repeat the cycle of contracting-releasing the muscles for 5-10 times.

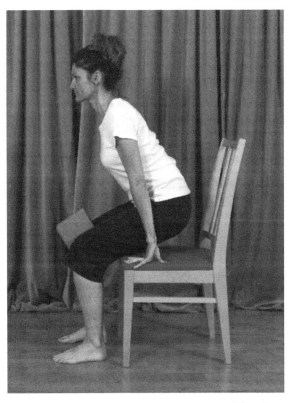

Figure 31: Chair pose with a block 1

If your legs are strong enough to support standing and walking, you may start working at a different level of intensity then the one suggested above (Chair pose with a block 2).

- Start standing about one foot, one foot and a half behind the chair, depending how long your arms are and how far forward you are going to angle the body. The feet are parallel and placed about pelvis distance apart for easier balance.

- Place the hands on the back of the chair keep the arms straight but do not lock in the elbows.

- Draw in from bellow the navel and slightly tuck the tailbone to engage the abdominal muscles. You should feel the pelvis slightly tilting toward the back. Breath naturally, without straining.

- Squat as you angle the torso forward. Maintain the weight predominantly on your heels.

- Go only as deep as you can maintain proper alignment: keep the back straight without arching, place the weight on the heels, keep the knees behind the toes even if not quite over the ankles, and the lower portion of the abdomen gently drawing in.

- Keep drawing in the navel and slightly tuck the tailbone to engage the abdominal muscles. You should feel the pelvis slightly tilting toward the back. Breath naturally, without straining.

- Squat as you angle the torso forward. Maintain the weight predominantly on your heels.

- Hold for 5 breath cycles at first, and then gradually increase the duration.

You can repeat the pose several times in a sequence or at different moments during the practice.

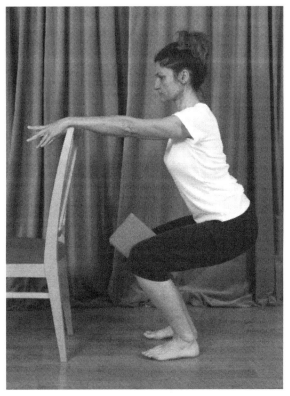

Figure 32: Chair pose with a block 2

3.8 Dancer Pose

Benefits

The pose stretches the front of the thigh muscles, improves knee flexibility by gently stretching the patellar tendon, stretches the major hip flexors and by doing this decompresses the lower back.

Technique

The Dancer pose can be approached differently according to one's own level of comfort with balance and flexibility of the knee joint. If your balance is uncertain and the ability to bend the knee quite limited then you should try the variation with one knee supported on the chair, as follows (see). Have the yoga strap or anything that you think you can use as replacement at hand.

- Start in standing position, facing the side of the chair with the left hand holding on the chair back.

- Bring the right knee on the chair with the hipbone vertical.

- Bend the knee further to grab the ankle with the right hand. If you cannot get the hand to hold on the ankle, then use the strap to extend the reach. Loop it around the ankle and hold as close to the foot as possible.

- Get the right foot closer to the rear end.

- Tuck the tailbone and engage the rear end muscles. You should feel the pelvis pressing forward and the front of the leg muscles stretching. If you feel too much intensity around the kneecap you should widen the angle at the knee by lessening the pull of the right foot.

- Hold for about 5 breath cycles.

- Do the other side.

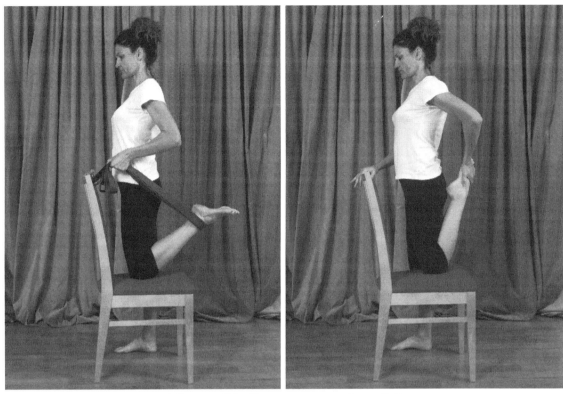

Figure 33: Dancer pose 1 and 2

There is a more challenging version of the *Dancer Pose* requiring better balance and slightly more flexibility in the knee joint (Figure 34: Dancer pose variation).

- Start standing behind the chair, about forearm distance away.

- Have the at hand.

- Hold on the chair back with your left hand keeping the elbow bend at about 90 degrees.

- Transfer the weight on the left leg.

- Bend the right knee. Take hold of your right ankle with the right hand. If you cannot reach then use the strap to hold your right ankle.

- Have the knees in line with each other and close together.

- Engage the rear end muscles and tuck the tailbone.

- Maintain the abdominals engaged by drawing in from bellow the navel.

- You should feel the pelvis pressing forward and the front of the leg muscles stretching. If you feel too much intensity around the kneecap you should widen the angle at the knee by lessening the pull of the right foot.

- Hold for about 5 breath cycles.

- Do the other side.

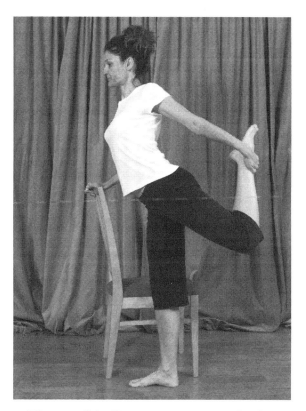

Figure 34: Dancer pose variation

3.9 Wide legged standing forward fold

Benefits

This pose is similar to the Standing forward fold but it also stretches the hamstrings in addition to the inner thighs and lower back muscles.

Technique

- Start standing in *Mountain pose* (see Figure 23) at about one, one and a half afoot in front of the chair, facing the seat.

- Set the feet parallel, about leg length apart.

- Inhale and lift the arms overhead.

- Exhale and fold forward, getting the hands on the seat with flat palms.

- Allow the arms to support the weight of the torso, still keeping some degree of softness in your shoulders, elbows and wrists.

- Drop the head, softening the back of the neck muscles.

- If you are flexible enough, you can place your forearms on the seat.

- In time you may become able to bring the forehead to the seat.

- If you are new to yoga and uncomfortable being head down, start by holding this position for 3 breathe cycles. As you are getting increasingly comfortable about it, you can extend the time up to 10 breaths cycles.

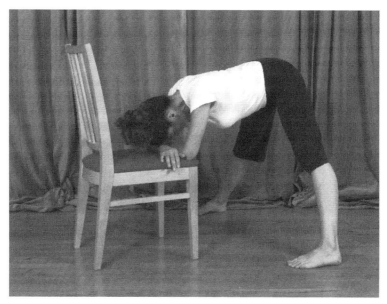

Figure 35: Wide-legged standing forward fold 1

3.10 Working deeper into the hip joint

This is a great way to enhance hip flexibility by increasing the hip joint lubrication and increase blood flow in the associated tissues (see Figure 36: Wide-legged standing forward fold 2). It helps preventing the formation of deposits and adhesions that in time would affect the functioning of the hip joint.

Technique

- Start in a wide legged standing forward fold with your hands placed on the seat (see Figure 34: Wide legged standing forward fold).

- You can keep the arms straight or flex the elbows slightly.

- Keep the neck relaxed.

- Keeping the knees straight, shift the pelvis side to side, "sinking" into the hop joints as you move. Go slowly. You don't have to follow the breath for this sequence.

- Do it about 10 times.

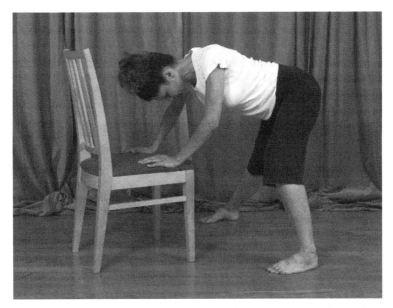

Figure 36: Wide-legged standing forward fold 2

3.11 Warrior 1

Benefits

This pose works toward strengthening the lower body and stretching the hip flexors. Since the largest among the hip flexors is connected to the lumbar spine and stretching it contributes to prevention or alleviating back pain.

Technique

- Start in *Mountain pose* (see Figure 23) facing the back of the chair, about one foot away.

- Rest the hands on the back support. The elbows should bend slightly.

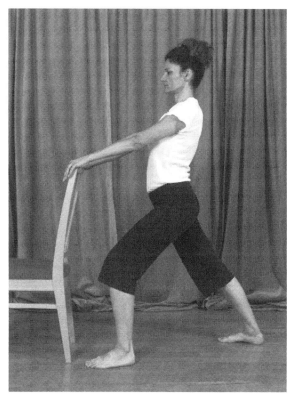

Figure 37: Warrior 1

- Set the feet parallel, about pelvis distance apart or slightly less.

- Step the right foot back slightly less then leg length.

- Bend the left knee.

- Keep the pelvis square; don't allow the right sight of your pelvis to get farther back then the left side.

- Ground the back foot flat on the floor with the toe angled in.

- Keep the back leg straight.

- Engage slightly the rear end muscles and stretch the tailbone down toward the ground to prevent the lower back from arching.

- Lift the breastbone to convey more length to the upper body.

- Keep the shoulders relaxed.

- Keep the jaw parallel to the floor.

- Gaze forward without straining the muscles in your face.

- Hold 5-10 breaths cycles, then come back to standing mountain.

- Do the other side.

3.12 Warrior 3

Benefits

This pose works on developing balance while it strengthens the core, legs and the upper back muscles.

Technique

- Start in *Mountain pose* (see Figure 23) facing the back of the chair, arm length away.

- Rest the hands on the back support. The elbows should be straight but not locked in.

- Set the feet parallel slightly less then pelvis distance apart.

- Maintain the left leg straight and place the weight on the left foot.

- Keep the pelvis parallel to the chair.

- Start hinging the torso forward while lifting the right leg behind.

- Keep the right ankle flexed.

- Have the head, neck, upper body and the right leg in a straight line. Don't angle the torso forward farther then you can lift your back leg.

- Keep the toes facing down.

- Drop the right side of the pelvis to be in line with the left.

- Your position may range from being slightly inclined forward (Figure 38: Warrior 3, Stage 1) to parallel to the floor (Figure 39: Warrior 3, Stage 2).

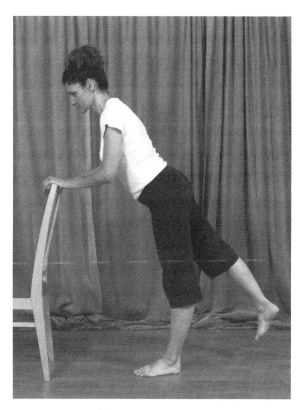

Figure 38: Warrior 3, Stage 1

- Hold 5-10 breaths cycles.

- Inhale and come back to Mountain pose (see Figure 23: Mountain pose).

• Do the other side.

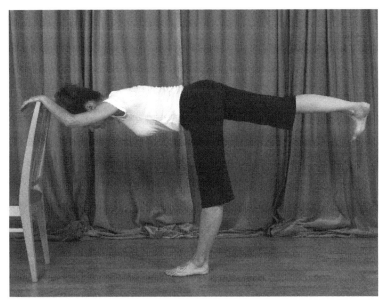

Figure 39: Warrior 3, Stage 2

3.13 Triangle

Benefits

This pose strengthen the legs and the back, stretches the inner thighs muscles, opens up the pelvis and the chest contributing to good posture and good breathing.

Technique

• Start in *Mountain pose* (see Figure 23) with the seat of the chair to your left side, about one, one a half foot away.

• Step your right foot to the right slightly less then leg length apart. Flexible persons can place the feet a full leg length apart.

• Turn your left toe out. Check for your front heel to be in line with the arch of your back foot.

- Keep the pelvis aligned to the wall in front of you, imagining that both pelvic bones could touch the wall simultaneously.

- Tuck the tailbone to keep a long spine in the lower back region.

- Lift the breastbone.

- Lengthen the neck.

- Stretch the arms out to the sides parallel to the floor.

- Look over your left fingertips.

- Keep the legs straight while sliding the hips to the right deepening the crease in your left hip.

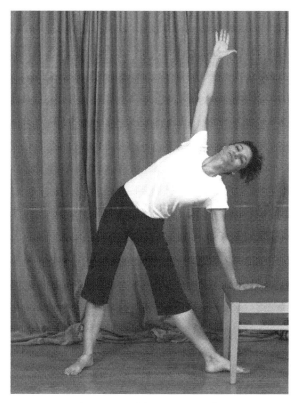

Figure 40: Triangle

- Tilt the torso sideway toward the chair maintaining equal length in both sides of the body. Do not allow your left side to round and shorten as you bend.

- Place the left arm on the seat to support the weight of the torso and assist balance.

- Stretch the right arm overhead. If this is problematic due to neck issues, support the hand on the right hip.

- You can allow the head to hang for a breath or two to stretch the neck muscles. Position the head in line with the rest of the body. You can keep the head neutral by keeping the left ear parallel to the floor, turn the face up, or look down.

- Hold for 5-10 breaths cycles.

- Bring the torso vertical and lower the arms.

- Step the feet together.

- Do the other side.

3.14 Standing Side Bend

Benefits

This pose works toward developing spine flexibility through side bending. It also stretches the intercostal muscles increasing the flexibility of the rib cage therefore enhancing breathing capacity (see Figure 41: Standing side bend).

Technique

- Start in *Mountain pose* (see Figure 23) with the seat of the chair to your left side, about one, one a half-foot away.

- Hold on the chair's back support with the left hand, but don't pull the chair toward you.

- Step the feet about 6 inches apart.

- Lift the right arm overhead. If you cannot lift the arm completely overhead go as high up as comfortable, without shrugging the shoulder and jam the neck. You can rest the hand on the waist if you cannot lift the arm due to shoulder injury, neck injury or any condition such as frozen shoulder.

- Slowly bend to the left, stretching the right side of the body. Go far enough to feel an engaging stretch but not so far to make breathing elaborate.

- Press the right foot firmly into the ground and lean into the right hip joint to stretch the outer leg as well.

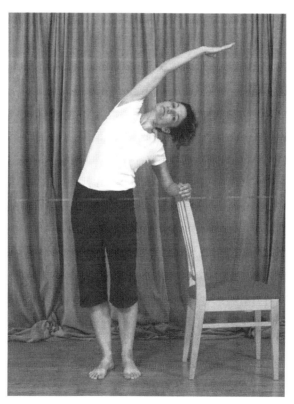

Figure 41: Standing side bend

- If you do have a hip replacement keep the pelvis centered. Don't allow the hips to slide to the right and keep the weight evenly distributed on both feet.

- Keep the neck neutral with the left ear parallel to the floor until you bend to the desired depth.

- Bend only as far as you can keep the back aligned to the wall behind. Imagine that both shoulder blades can touch the wall behind simultaneously.

- You may look up to challenge the neck muscles and the upper body.

- You may look down if you need to protect the neck.

- Come back vertical then pause in *Mountain* pose.

- Do the other side.

- Hold 3-5 breath cycles per each side.

3.15 Crescent pose

Benefits

This pose is similar in many aspects to *Warrior 1*. It makes it easier to keep the pelvis square since the back heel is not grounded yet it challenges the balance because the back heel is off the ground. Same as *Warrior 1* (see Figure 37), it works toward strengthening the lower body and stretching the hip flexors. Stretching the hip flexors helps prevent or alleviate back pain related to stiffness in these muscles.

Technique

- Start in *Mountain pose* (see Figure 23) facing the back of the chair, about one foot away.

- Rest the hands on the back support. The elbows should straight but not locked in.

- Set the feet parallel, about pelvis distance apart or slightly less.

- Step the right foot back about leg length.

- Bend the left knee.

- Keep the pelvis square; don't allow the right sight of your pelvis to get farther back then the left side.

- Keep the ball of your back foot on the floor with. The heel remains up.

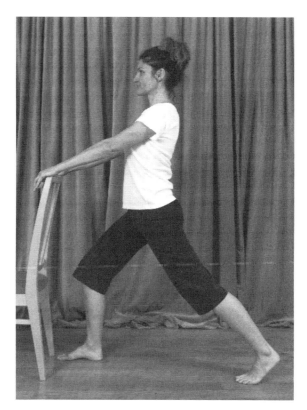

Figure 42: Crescent pose

- Bend the back knee; tuck the tailbone until you feel your pelvis getting leveled to the ground. Keep the pelvis level and stretch the back leg the best you can.

- Engage slightly the rear end muscles and stretch the tailbone down toward the ground to prevent the lower back from arching.

- Lift the breastbone to convey more length to the upper body.

- Keep the shoulders relaxed.

- Keep the jaw parallel to the floor.

- Gaze forward without straining the muscles in your face.

- Lighten the support from your hands and allow the legs and core muscles to take over.

- Hold 5-10 breaths cycles.

- To come out use the hands for full support if you need, then lift the pelvis a little widening the angle in your front knee. Step the back foot forward.

- With the hands still on the chair bend slightly both knees, allow the back to soften and round, then get vertical by rolling the spine up one vertebra at a time. The head is the last one to move up. When you completed the transition come back to *Mountain pose*.

- Do the other side.

3.16 High Lounge

Benefits

High Lounge position brings in a bit more strengthening work for the abdominals in addition to focus on balance and legs strengthening and stretching. Since it does not require a back bent, it can be used as a substitute for *Crescent pose* (see Figure 42) whenever back bends are not well suited.

Technique

This pose is similar in many ways to the *Crescent Pose* and *Warrior 1*. It makes it easier to keep the pelvis square since the back heel is not grounded yet it challenges the balance because the back heel is off the ground. Same as *Warrior 1*, it works toward strengthening the lower body and stretching the hip flexors. Since the largest among the hip flexors is connected to the lumbar spine, it may cause back pain if left un-stretched.

- Start in *Mountain pose* (see Figure 23) facing the front of the chair (the seat), about one foot away.

- Rest the hands on the seat support. The elbows should straight, but not locked in.

- Set the feet parallel, about pelvis distance apart or slightly less.

- Step the right foot back about leg length while bending slightly the left knee.

- Before lounging any deeper, make sure your left knee is over the ankle and not past the toes. Keep the lower leg perpendicular on the floor. Also, tuck slightly the tailbone and draw in from bellow the navel to engage the abdominals, supporting the lower back.

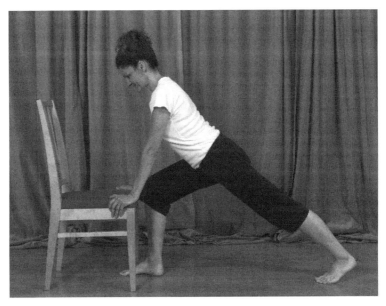

Figure 43: High lounge

- Keep the pelvis square; don't allow the right sight of your pelvis to get farther back then the left side.

- Get the back leg straight by pressing the heel away.

- Gaze about one foot in front, maintaining the neck neutral.

- Lounge as deep as you wish without giving up any alignment details you've got in place. Feel the head, the neck, the upper body and the back leg from hip joint to the back heal forming in one straight line.

- If you want more intensity in this position lessen the amount of support on your hands; get really light on your palms allowing all the muscles in the body to take over.

- Hold for 5-10 breath cycles.

- To come out use the hands for full support if you need, then lift the pelvis a little widening the angle in your front knee. Step the back foot forward.

- With the hands still on the chair bend slightly both knees, allow the back to soften and round, then get vertical by rolling the spine up one vertebra at a time. The head is the last one to move upright. When you completed the transition come back to *Mountain pose.*

- Do the other side

4 Restorative poses

Restorative poses are easy poses, very gentle on the body but their impact on physiology is deep. Modern science speaks more and more about the neuromuscular system as opposed to treat the muscular system separately from the nervous system because the two are deeply interconnected, so working with one triggers a reaction into the other. By allowing the muscles to rest in a position that is very comfortable still providing good alignment, the nervous system also relaxes and the neurotransmitters responsible for feeling deeply relaxed, calm, and happy are released into the bloodstream. You can learn more about restorative yoga from Judith Laseter's *Relax and Renew* book (Laseter, 1995).

4.1 Supported seated forward fold

Benefits

The pose promotes relaxation of the neck and back muscles and a very mild, soft stretch in hamstrings.

Technique

This pose requires the use of some props, such as a pillow wrapped in a blanket in addition to the chair and the block and/or books recommended for feet support. If you don't have a pillow at hand, then wrap one or two foam blocks in a yoga blanket or beach towel to make a thick bolster.

- Place the feet on blocks or stack of books to get the thighs level to the ground or about an inch higher then the seat. This prevents the bolster from sliding away.

- Place the bolster on your lap and curl around it.

- Cross the arms on top and support your forehead.

- Close the eyes.

- Hold for at least 10 breath cycles.

- Come out of the pose slowly.

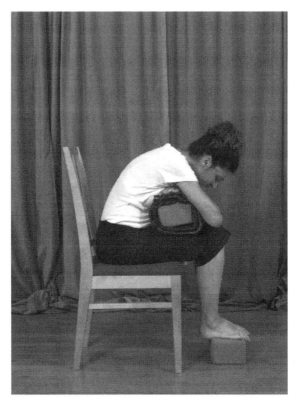

Figure 44: Supported seated forward fold

4.2 Supported seated side bend

Benefits

This pose allows for deep relaxation while opening and stretching mildly one side of the body.

Technique

- Sit sideway on the chair with your left side touching the back support.

- Make a bolster by wrapping one or two blocks in a blanket or beach towel. The bolster should be thinner then the one used for the *Seated forward fold* otherwise it will take too much space off the seat.

- Squeeze the bolster between your left side and the back of the chair.

- Place the left arm and forearm on top of the back support. Place the right hand on the back support, too.

- Bend to the left over the bolster and rest the head on your left forearm and your right hand. The head may be leaning on one the side with the left ear parallel to the floor or you may turn the face down and support the forehead.

- Close the eyes.

- Hold for at least 7 breath cycles.

- Come out of the pose slowly.

- Do the other side.

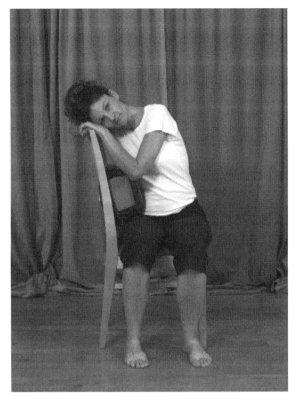

Figure 45: Supported seated side bend

4.3 Deep resting pose at the end of the practice

Benefits

This pose allows your nervous system to rest deeply and helps the body assimilate the benefits of the whole practice.

Technique

- This pose completes the practice by allowing the body to sink

- Support the legs on blocks or a stack of books to relief the pooling of blood and lymph in your lower legs occurring from long hours of standing or seat with the lower legs hanging down.

- Sit with the back supported without slouching. You may place a small bolster behind the middle and lower back. This is more doable if seated on an office chair or airplane seat. It may not be suitable for folding chairs, which are most commonly used for chair yoga practice since they have a gap in the correspondence of the lower back. If you use a folding chair cushion the back with blankets before adding the bolster. If you can lean back and relax without

- Place a rolled beach towel on top of your shoulders behind your neck to support the head. The thicker the roll the more support will provide.

- For the first 2-5 minutes, depending on how long you intend to be in this pose, you can do one of the following *Complete breathing*, *Step breathing 1 and 2*, or *Alternate nostril breathing* described in *Chapter 6*.

- You can practice this position by itself at anytime you feel the need for some deep rest and circumstances that don't allow for a longer nap. You can also use it in combination with the guided relaxation presented below.

- If you use the pose in combination with breathing or guided relaxation make sure to spent about 5 minutes of plain silence in addition to the time spent with breathing practice and/or that allotted to the guided relaxation before you come out.

- If thoughts are coming, don't entertain them, don't pause or focus on any of them, simply allow thoughts to flow through.

- You may set a timer so you can relax without minding the time.

- Come out slowly; don't jump off the chair because this is counterproductive.

- If your coming out of the *Deep resting pose* is too sudden you may experience unpleasant things going on, such as being irritable, notice your heart rate increasing occasionally, and not feel rested and refreshed at all. Not allowing enough time to transition would be the equivalent of a bucket of cold water being dumped on you while asleep! How soothing and calming would that feel?

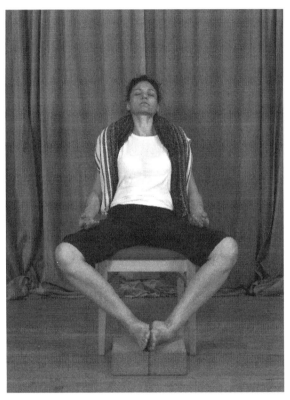

Figure 46: Deep resting pose

5 Guided Relaxation

5.1 Benefits

This guided relaxation complements the *Deep resting pose* (Figure 46). The guided relaxation involves intentional mental activity in form as visualization and body awareness, while the *Deep resting pose* is all about mental silence and non-thinking. When doing the *Guided relaxation* followed by another five minutes in the *Deep resting pose*, the effect of the of whole practice becomes more powerful. You will experience more energy, mental clarity and an increased sense of overall wellbeing.

You can learn by heart this meditation and then mentally give yourself guidance as you go through it.

5.2 Technique

- Start in the *Deep resting pose* (see Figure 46).

- Close the eyes.

- Breath relaxed at your normal pace, inhaling and exhaling through the nose.

- Observe the breath as it flows smoothly through the body. Just observe it without trying to influence it in anyway.

- Now focus on the exhalation.

- Feel every exhalation as it comes from the depth of your body and flows out through the nose removing tension in your muscles, organs, cleaning all the physical, mental and emotional debris.

- Feel the exhalation removing the tension in the lower legs, and the lower legs are getting lighter and softer.

- Feel the exhalation removing the tension in the upper legs, and the upper legs are getting lighter and softer.

- Feel the exhalation removing the tension in the pelvis, and the pelvic area is getting lighter and softer.

- Feel the exhalation removing the tension in your abdomen, and your abdomen is getting lighter and softer.

- Feel the exhalation removing the tension in your chest, and feel chest getting lighter and softer.

- Feel the exhalation removing the tension in your neck, and feel the neck getting lighter and softer.

- Feel the exhalation removing the tension in your arms, and feel the arms getting lighter and softer.

- Feel the exhalation removing the tension in your head, the skull and the face, and feel the skull getting lighter and the face muscles getting softer.

- Visualize the air you exhale as a light bluish-grey vapors.

- With every exhalation the whole body is getting lighter and softer.

- It almost feels like dematerializing.

- Now focus on the inhalation.

- Feel inhalation moving in through the nostrils and flowing into the body.

- Visualize the air you breath in as a brilliant golden flow.

- Imagine your body as a tall vessel getting filled up with the brilliant golden flow pouring in with every exhale.

- Visualize the legs filling up with golden light from the toes up to the knees, and strength and vitality in your legs

- Visualize the thighs filling up with golden light from the knees up to the hip joints, and feel strength and vitality in your thighs.

- Visualize the pelvis filling up with golden light, and feel strength and vitality in your pelvis.

- Visualize the abdomen filling up with golden light, and feel strength and vitality in your abdominal region.

- Visualize the chest filling up with golden light, and feel strength and vitality in your chest.

- Visualize the neck filling up with golden light, and feel strength and vitality in your neck and throat.

- Visualize the arms filling up with golden light from the fingertips up to the shoulders, and feel strength and vitality in your arms.

- Visualize the head filling up with golden light, and feel strength and vitality in your skull, your brain and your face.

- Feel every inhalation nourishing and energizing your entire being.

- Feel every exhalation cleansing and relaxing.

- Visualize the air you breath in as a brilliant golden flow.

- Visualize the air you exhale as thin, light bluish-grey vapors.

- ...breath-in a brilliant golden flow.

- ...breath out thin, light bluish grey vapors.

- Breath deeper, with increased awareness of the breath.

- Keep the eyes closed and become more aware of your own body.

- Expand the awareness to the chair you are sitting on, and to the space of the room you are in.

- Start moving slowly.

- One more deep breath-in, and exhale with a rewarding "Aaaaahhhhh!"

- Smile big and slowly open the eyes.

- Have a wonderful rest of the day!

6 Breathing Practice

Breathing is important because breathing patterns affect physiology. In other words the way we breathe influences or mood, our overall health, our performance (Iyengar, Light on Life: The Yoga Journey to Wholeness, Inner Peace, and Ultimate Freedom, 2005). Here are few aspects of breathing worthy of consideration.

6.1 Chest breathing

Many people are chest breathers, which means that only their chest expands with the inhale and recedes with the exhale. The abdomen is usually immobile, looking and feeling lifeless. Sometimes the collarbones are visibly moving up and down with the breath. The breath is shallow and rapid. Such people are usually tense, snappy, angry, feeling constantly stressed or pressured. They seem unable to relax. Common ailments in chest breathers are high blood pressure, ulcer, asthma, anxiety, and depression. Chest breathing stimulates predominantly the sympathetic nervous system that is responsible for the "fight or flight" response, hence answer about the relationship between chest breathing and ailments known as stress related.

Another deficiency of chest breathing is under using the lungs capacity. The lungs are breathing organs located inside the ribcage. They are narrower at the top and wider at the bottom. Chest breathing will act predominantly upon the top portion of the lungs a leaving the bottom portion mostly unused. In these circumstances the intake of air is very limited, the oxygen intake is much reduced with detrimental effects on the brain, heart, and other vital organs.

6.2 Abdominal breathing

Abdominal breathing is the natural complement for chest breathing. Strictly speaking, abdominal breathing alone does not exist, but there may be a predominance of the abdominal wall moving with the breath. People displaying a balance between chest and belly moving with the breath, breathing slowly and deeper are usually in a better state of balance, calmer and more resilient to stress, therefore less prone to stress related conditions. Abdominal breathing stimulates the parasympathetic nervous system that is responsible for the "rest and digest" mode. Its role is that of calming nerves following overstimulation and enhances digestion. Abdominal breathing acts upon the bottom portion of the allowing for increased air intake and better oxygenation.

Abdominal and chest breathing are both components of natural, complete and healthy breathing. Because the physiological act of breathing has a profound effect on the nervous system balancing breath leads to balancing the activity of parasympathetic and sympathetic nervous systems. Below is a suggested practice to cultivate healthy breathing habits.

6.3 Complete breathing

Benefits

Complete breathing works toward balancing the sympathetic and parasympathetic nervous system, exercises the intercostal muscles, enhances the lungs functioning.

Technique

You can practice complete breathing as often as you wish during the day, at any time. You can do it in the beginning of your yoga practice or throughout it in association with any of the seated, standing or restorative poses.

Chest breathing practice

- Sit comfortably on the chair. You can sit with back support but don't slouch.

- Place one hand on the chest and one hand on the abdomen.

- Inhale, expanding the chest only. You should feel the hand on the chest rising with the inhale while the hand on the abdomen remains steady.

- Exhale, releasing the chest only. Feel the hand on the chest descending with the exhale while the hand on the belly remains steady.

- Do 3-5 cycles of chest breathing.

Abdominal breathing practice

- Inhale, expanding only the belly. You should feel the hand on the belly rising with the inhale while the hand on the chest remains steady.

- Exhale, releasing the abdomen. Feel the hand on the abdomen descending with the exhale while the hand on the chest remains steady.

- Do 3-5 cycles of abdominal breathing.

Complete breathing practice

- Inhale expanding first the abdomen and then the chest. You should feel the hand on the belly rising firs on the beginning of the inhale then the hand on the chest following as your inhale progresses.

- Exhale, releasing the chest and the abdomen simultaneously.

- Do at least 10 cycles of complete breathing.

6.4 Lengthening the exhale

Benefits

Learning to control the duration of your exhale is a very good exercise that enhances the lung capacity and lower the heart rate.

Technique

- Sit comfortably on the chair. You can sit with back support but don't slouch.

- Take a full inhale. The inhale should be complete, but not forced. Asses how many counts does it take for you to inhale.

- Exhale on the same number of counts.

- Do this a couple of times, inhaling and exhaling on the same number of counts. (Let's say a count of 6 /inhale + a count of 6 /exhale).

- Take a full inhale (let's say a count of 6) and make the exhale one count longer (count of 7 in this example)

- Take a full inhale (let's say a count of 6) and make the exhale two counts longer (count of 8 in this example)

- Progress until your exhale gets to be one and a half times longer then the inhale (count of 9 in this example). Don't strain, and give yourself time to reach this step. It may take several days to achieve it. Practice at the level you feel comfortable and built up intensity gently and gradually.

- Do at least 10 cycles at your current level of ability.

6.5 Breath of Fire

Benefits

This type of breathing energizes and builds heat in the body in a very gentle way. It also helps maintaining the focus on the practice.

Technique

- Sit comfortably on the chair with the back upright and unsupported.

- Rest the hands on the lap.

- You can practice with the eyes closed or open.

- Narrow slightly the wind pipes in such way that the air will move in and out with a slight hissing sound due to the friction of the air flow against the narrowed throat.

- The sound should be soft, and loud enough for you to hear but not so loud to be heard from across the room. Trying to get it sound louder may irritate the throat and make it soar.

- If you don't feel comfortable to inhale with the throat constricted, do *Breath of Fire* on exhale alone and inhale as you would breathe normally.

6.6 Breathing in Steps

Benefits

This breathing practice has two parts that balance each other. Inhaling in steps is gently energizing and warming while exhaling in steps is calming and cooling. You can practice the two parts separately at different times of the day, or together as a single exercise.

Technique

Part 1

- Sit comfortably on the chair with the back upright and unsupported.

- Take a deep inhale, then exhale completely.

- Inhale one third of your total capacity and hold the breath for two seconds.

- Inhale the second third of your total capacity and hold the breath for two seconds.

- Inhale the last third of your total capacity and hold the breath for two seconds.

- Exhale smoothly and completely.

- Do 5 rounds or more.

Part 2

- Take full inhale.

- Exhale one third of your total capacity and hold the breath for two seconds.

- Exhale the second third of your total capacity and hold the breath for two seconds.

- Exhale the last third of your total capacity and hold the breath out for two seconds.

- Inhale smoothly and completely.

- Do 5 rounds or more.

6.7 Alternate nostril breathing

Benefits

This breathing practice helps balancing right and left side of the brain, balances the energy flow in the body, improves concentration, enhances awareness, and induces a state of calmness (see Figure 47: Alternate nostril breathing).

Technique

- Sit comfortably on the chair with the back upright and preferably unsupported.

- If you have to use back support, don't slouch.

- Traditionally the right thumb and the ring finger are used for this practice.

- Open your right hand.

- Fold the index and the middle finger into your palm, separating the thumb from the ring finger and the pinky.

- If you don't feel comfortable with this positioning of the fingers, then use any two fingers from your right hand (thumb and index, for example).

- Bring the right hand in front of the face with fingers in the position described above.

- Occlude the right nostril by pressing with the thumb on the outside.

- Inhale through the left nostril.

- Occlude the left nostril by pressing the ring finger (or index if you've chosen the simpler way to position the hand) and release the right nostril.

- Exhale through the right nostril.

- Inhale through the right nostril.

- Occlude the right nostril with the thumb and release the left.

- Exhale through the left nostril.

- This counts as one breath cycle

- Do at least 5 cycles.

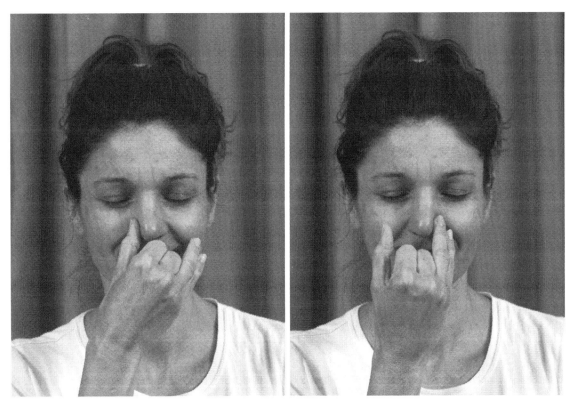

Figure 47: Alternate nostril breathing

7 Leverage Your Potential

Everything that reaches our person in the form of food, clothing, makeup, TV programs, people we interact with, has an impact on our health, for better or for worse. We need to become aware what old habits are detrimental to our health and limit our potential, and what new habits we can adopt to leverage our potential and better our health.

Modern life brings the *freedom* to choose from a variety of lifestyles and habits, and it also brings the *responsibility* to choose wisely among them. Humans evolved over several hundred thousands years and our genes learned to adapt to small changes over a lifetime. In the last few hundred years, we brought explosive changes in our lifestyle, which, chosen without discrimination, could break down the ability of our genes and immune system to adapt. The book *Nutrition and Physical Degeneration* (Price, 2008) is just one example of how modern nutrition could impact our health. Fortunately, it is possible to reverse degenerative diseases by undoing some of the unhealthy choices that the western world adopted lately, and especially in the last hundred years. As Socrates said, "the unexamined life is not worth living", since we may end up repeating the same mistakes that our ancestors did. Yet, changing habits is hard and it takes a lot of perseverance to be successful.

The material presented in the previous chapters addresses primarily the musculo-skeletal system. Some postures, such as twists and forward folds, work on the internal organs as well, providing a gentle massage, in particular of bowels, liver and kidneys. We can leverage the benefits of our yoga practice and increase the rate of our progress by making conscious choices about lifestyle and nutrition.

7.1   We Are What We Think

Iyengar (Iyengar, 2005) reminds us that in order to achieve a serene consciousness, a prerequisite for success in life, we need to change our behavior and approach toward the external world:

> *"If you are happy, pleasant, and unselfish in your behavior towards others, obstacles will shrink. If you are miserly with your emotions and judgmental in your mind, obstacles will grow."*

In his *Goals* book (Tracy, 2003), Brian Tracy uncovers that we become what we think most of the time. Thoughts lead to actions, actions lead to habits, and habits determine our destiny. Og Mandino (Mandino, 1983) shows us how we can leverage habits to change significant aspects of our life:

> *"Good habits are the key to all success. Bad habits are the unlocked door to failure. Thus, the first law I will obey which precedeth all others – I will form good habits and become their slave."*

Dr. Schultze (Schultze, 2010) expresses the same idea as follows:

> *"Getting well is just a matter of stopping what you did to make yourself sick and beginning a few new programs that will encourage health."*

For example, fear makes us think, most of the time, at what we do not want and, as a consequence, prevents us to attract what we want in our life. A positive attitude is essential for our success in any endeavor, including health. And if we are afraid of something, such as bad health, we can do something that makes the fear disappear, such as exercise more and improve our diet. The challenge is to build our motivation and desire to change, which can be accomplished using the methods outlined in Section 1.3.

7.2 We Are What We Eat

Water and fresh juices

Clean filtered water is a prerequisite for removing toxins from our bodies to help rejuvenating us. Fresh vegetables and low-glycemic fruit juices (such as carrots, beets, green apples) provide vitamin, minerals and especially enzymes, in a form easy to assimilate even for sick people. Everything else, including sodas and alcoholic beverages are a burden for our elimination systems (Schultze, 2010). A water filter, such as activated charcoal or reverse osmosis, is essential to provide clean, pure water to our bodies. A juicer is essential to provide fresh juices to your diet. Pasteurized juices, commonly found in food stores, lack enzymes, since the pasteurization process destroys them (Cousens, 2003). According to Dr. Cousens and Dr. Schultze, bringing fresh juices in your diet leverages the rejuvenating processes at cellular level.

Whole foods and seaweeds

In the book *In Defense of Food: An Eater's Manifesto* (Pollan, 2009), Michael Pollan summarizes a healthy attitude towards foods:

"Eat food. Not too much. Mostly plants".

By "food" we mean traditional whole foods, processed minimally to preserve their vitamins, minerals and enzymes. Organic fruits and vegetables are recommended due to their higher vitamin and mineral content. Seaweeds provide additional minerals, such as iodine, that complement organically grown fruits and vegetables (Wigmore, 1983).

Rainbow-green Live-food Cuisine (Cousens, 2003) provides a delicious collection of vegan meals, which may support your quest for improving your health. While not everyone has to become a raw-food vegan, increasing the quantity of raw and fermented vegetables, low-glycemic fruits (such as berries and green apples), sprouted nuts and beans, and fresh juices has the ability provide vitamins, minerals, enzymes and fiber in a bio-available form, which are essential for a healthy life-style. And a fresh juice fast, using juices made in your own juicer, can do wonders for your health. For more details about juice fasting and its benefits, we suggest Dr. Schultze's *20 Steps for Powerful Health* (Schultze, 2010), available online at www.herbdocblog.com.

7.3 Be persistent!

It takes about three to six months of continuous practice for a routine to be firmly established, so being constant in practicing your newly acquired skills is a must. Expect obstacles and setbacks on your path but don't get discouraged. An unexpected trip or illness may upset your schedule. Don't make excuses to take a brake from your newly established habits but also, don't get frustrated and even more important, don't beat yourself up when you really have to back off for a short while. Whenever this happens, just come back to your practice. Be prepared to come back one hundred times, if necessary remembering that the journey is more important then the destination. While addressing a young audience, Sir Winston Churchill summarized the lessons of his life in seven words:

"Never give up. Never, never give up!"

Resources

Yoga Props

YogaAccessories.com (www.yogaaccessories.com) is a source of quality yoga props (blankets, straps, blocks), equipment and supplies at wholesale prices.

Manduka (http://www.manduka.com) offers high performance yoga products (mats, straps, blocks) and yoga gear.

Whole Unrefined Foods

Whole Foods Market (http://www.wholefoodsmarket.com) sells high quality natural and organic products. Use it as a guide to improve your eating habits.

Seaweeds

Maine Coast Sea Vegetables (https://www.seaveg.com) specializes in sustainably harvested seaweeds, such as Dulse and Kelp. They are rich in minerals, such as iodine, usually not found in land vegetables. Seaweeds in granules and powder forms can be sprinkled in salads or mixed in smoothies, while whole leafs can be used in Miso soup.

Herbs

Pacific Botanicals (http://www.pacificbotanicals.com) sells wholesale only organically grown and wild-harvested herbs.

iHerb.com (http://www.iherb.com) provides natural products, including herbs in bulk, at significant discount prices. Some of our family's favorites include:

- *Organic Green Power Blend* by Starwest Botanicals is high in chlorophyll, antioxidants, minerals, vitamins and enzymes.

- *Brewer's Yeast* (grown on beet molasses) by Modern Products or Lewis Labs is high in B vitamins, minerals and amino acids.

- *Organic Rosehips Powder* by Starwest Botanicals is high in C vitamin. You can make your own natural multi mineral and vitamin formula by mixing the above three complementary ingredients in desired proportions. Be creative and add other ingredients as well. Just sprinkle it in your own made vegetable juices, smoothies and salads for an incredible boost in energy.

- *Quick Colon Formula* (Part 1 and Part 2) by Christopher's Original Formula. Remember, if we do not have two bowel movements per day, we are constipated. Constipation facilitates both the production of toxins in the colon and their subsequent reabsorption in the bloodstream (Schultze, 2010).

- *Flax Oil* by Barleans for the essential Omega 3 oils.

- *Organic Extra Virgin Coconut Oil* by Nutiva is our first choice for cooking oil.

- *Organic Curry Powder by* Starwest Botanicals has many health benefits. Its main ingredient, turmeric, has antiseptic, antioxidant and anti-inflammatory properties.

Dr. Schulze (https://www.herbdoc.com) offers several outstanding natural healing programs (foundational, detox, specific). Free educational resources for natural healing, describing these programs, are available at Dr. Schulze's blog (https://herbdocblog.com).

Tree of Life Rejuvenation Center (http://www.treeoflife.nu/) is one of the top yoga and rejuvenation centers in the world. Led by Dr. Gabriel Cousens, M.D., the Center offers excellent holistic programs, most of them described in Dr. Cousens' books.

Kitchen Tools

Blenders

Vitamix (http://www.vitamix.com) offers high performance blenders, which provide an easy and delicious way to increase the quantity of vegetables and fruits in your diet. Blending increases digestibility and preserves enzymes, while the increased fiber content improves regularity.

Juicers

According to Dr. Schulze, drinking fresh juices is like a blood transfusion, rapidly restoring the quality of the blood even in anemic patients. I recommend mostly masticating juicers, as opposed to high-speed centrifugal juicers, since they avoid oxidation and preserve better the quality of the juices. You can really taste the difference. The juicers below are also better at juicing green vegetables, including wheatgrass. For juicer comparisons please check YouTube (http://www.youtube.com) and choose your favorite.

- **Green Star GS-1000** (http://www.greenstar.com) is a versatile juicer and food processor, which produces high quality juice.

- **Omega Vert VRT350HD** (http://www.omegajuicers.com) is a revolutionary high efficiency juicer in a compact vertical design.

- **Champion** (http://www.championjuicer.com) is an old-timer favorite. Make sure that you also get the "Greens Attachment" for juicing leafy greens and wheatgrass.

Bibliography

Coulter, H. D. (2001). *Anatomy of Hatha Yoga.* Body and Breath, Inc.

Cousens, G. (2003). *Rainbow Green Live-Food Cuisine.* North Atlantic Books.

Iyengar, B. (2005). *Light on Life: The Yoga Journey to Wholeness, Inner Peace, and Ultimate Freedom.* Rodale Books.

Iyengar, B. (2001). *Yoga: The Path to Holistic Health.* Great Britain: Dorling Kindersley Ltd.

Laseter, J. (1995). *Relax and Renew.* Berkeley, CA: Rodmell Press.

Mandino, O. (1983). *The Greatest Salesman in the World.* Bantam.

Pollan, M. (2009). *In Defense of Food .* Penguin.

Price, W. (2008). *Nutrition and Physical Degeneration.* Price Pottenger Nutrition.

Schiffman, E. (1996). *Yoga: The Spirit and Practice of Moving Into Stillness.* New York, NY: Pocket Books.

Schultze, R. (2010). *20 Powerful Steps to a Healthier Life.* Marina del Rey, CA: Natural Healing Publications (https://herbdocblog.com/).

Tracy, B. (2003). *Goals!: How to Get Everything You Want-Faster Than You Ever Thought Possible.* Berrett-Koehler Publishers.

Wigmore, A. (1983). *The Hippocrates Diet and Health Program.* Avery Trade.

Index

Made in the USA
Charleston, SC
12 January 2012